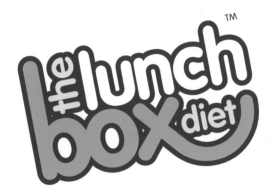

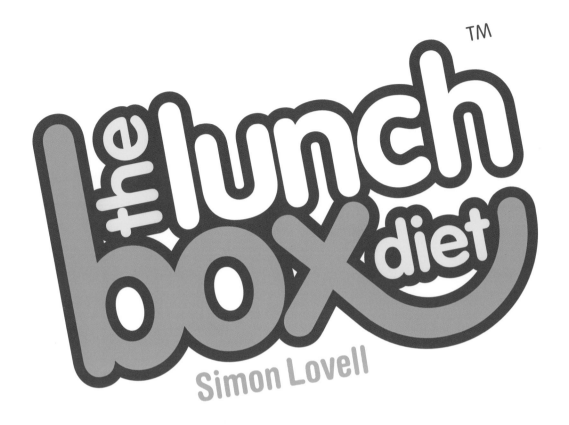

the lunch box diet ™

Simon Lovell

EAT ALL DAY, LOSE WEIGHT, FEEL GREAT

HarperCollins*Publishers*

HarperCollins*Publishers*
77–85 Fulham Palace Road,
Hammersmith, London W6 8JB

www.harpercollins.co.uk

First published by HarperCollins*Publishers* in 2009

10 9 8 7 6 5 4 3 2

Photographs © Mark Read
Home economy: Bethany Heald

The Lunch Box Diet branding:
Creative Gain, www.creativegain.co.uk

A catalogue record of this book is
available from the British Library

ISBN-13 978-0-00-728835-2

Printed and bound in Italy by
Rotolito, Lombarda SpA, Milan

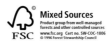

Contents

Acknowledgements

Crikey blimey, I never thought I'd have to write one of these acknowledgements pages so I feel very privileged. Where do I start? Of course – I want to thank HarperCollins for publishing this book and allowing the Lunch Box Diet to benefit so many more people than found it via the internet.

Thanks to Nicola Ibison at First Artists. Then there's my book agent, Luigi Bonomi of Bonomi Associates, who has been great throughout this whole process, as has Simon Gain at Creative Gain for helping me to develop the fantastic friendly branding. I'd also like to thank Vicky Stoakes and the crew at Indigo Cow PR – you have been and continue to be amazing – and Liz Mills at Top TV Academy for helping me develop my TV career. And thanks to Jamie Oliver for allowing me to help show (on *Jamie Saves Our Bacon*) how important it is that the animals we eat are treated as humanely as possible. It was hard, but very rewarding!

A bit closer to home now, and I can safely say that this book wouldn't be in your hands if it wasn't for the hard work of one man called Paul Christopher, or 'Barty', of Exesight Photography, who has been a friend of mine since primary school. We ran our own magazine and were generally known as the computer geeks.

To Nick Trent – you're a fantastic design talent and thank you so much for all your hard work on the original ebook.

To my friends, all of you (and your little sprogs) – you know who you are – thanks for being great and spurring me along when things have been tough. It makes a hell of a difference.

Cheers to all my work colleagues who make my days in the gym such fun and, of course, my clients. I love working with them and helping them to reach their goals.

Finally to Mum and Dad – what can I say? You've always given me that extra push that I've needed and enabled me to do things I would never have been able to do without your help. You are loved dearly.

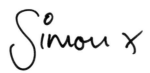

The Secret's in the Box

Repeat after me: Let my wobbly belly never fall below my waistline again. On this path, despite previous efforts, I shall not be stressed, hungry, count my calories or make silly meals. I have broken from the unhealthy grasp of eating only meat, sipping water, munching a lonely carrot, spooning baby food, cabbage soup or any other unsustainable fix. From this day forward I shall live life, be vibrant and energised. When I reach my goal I will stand tall, proud and full of zest and share with others, as they look on with envy, the words: 'The secret's in the box.'

First of all, well done!
Put a massive smile
on your face and feel
the energy flowing
from this second
onwards!

Chapter 1

Why the Lunch Box Diet?

The Lunch Box Diet is going to change the way you think about food, you'll learn to know your body better than you have ever done before and the benefits to you over the next days, weeks and years are going to be significant.

This diet won't only help you to lose weight; it might also get you doing more exciting things in your life. Maybe you'll change your job and dump that annoying boss? Before I expand on this I want to tell you more about me so we can start building our relationship, which is going to be very important to your success.

I've worked as a personal trainer for many clients in one of the largest health clubs in the UK, so I know how difficult it can be for busy people to eat a healthy diet. Day in, day out, I've coached everyone from stay-at-home mums and dads to busy office workers and sportsmen and -women and I've found that they all have different routines, which makes controlling food intake different for everyone.

I've learned that a lot of the diet plans out there only take into account the food on the plate, not the tough demands upon your time and mental energies that modern life can bring. Many diets involve preparing meals and adding ingredients you just wouldn't normally pick up, let alone have the time to prepare. My aim is to teach you how to build the Lunch Box Diet into your working day and train your taste buds to get used to a healthier way of eating. We'll work hard together and, with my support, you'll be able to get in shape, look great and feel more energised. It's not just good for losing weight; it can also help to sustain a healthy balance in your diet. If you're already an active person looking for an eating plan that complements your gym time, this plan will be ideal for you. This is the diet where you control what you eat based on your energy levels. What's more you'll never be hungry – ever – and you'll lose weight. Yep, keep smiling!

'The Lunch Box Diet is going to change the way you think about food'

My Story

I think it's very important that professionals who set out to teach other people should base their teaching on personal experience. I haven't been lean, strong and confident all my life – in fact, the contrary is true.

I was overweight in my early twenties and was easily a few jean sizes over what is classed as 'normal' these days. My average daily diet consisted of fried food, pizzas and microwave meals. My snacks were chocolate bars, my energy levels low and my confidence almost non-existent. When you're down there, it's hard to see out. I never thought that one day I would be writing a book about eating properly and spending most of my days teaching people how fitness and health can change their world. Hell, no!

But everyone has a turning point in their lives and mine came when I was bullied at school. Enough was enough. I joined a kung-fu class. At the class I met a guy called Tim. He took me under his wing, threw me into the gym and got me lifting weights. My body shape started to change and I got the buzz. I started attracting more girls – fantastic! As a guy who used to be the butt of everyone's jokes, I loved it. Who wouldn't? To Tim, who took me through those important first steps – thank you. I wouldn't be writing this now and helping others if you hadn't paid special attention to me.

Some of this back story may resonate with you because of experiences in your own life. It might not. But a lot of people who have problems with their weight have a story to tell. If I can connect with some of you in this way then we have a better chance of moving forward and developing together.

The Birth of the Diet

What I have found most satisfying about this project is that I never sat down and said, 'I'm going to write a diet plan.' It just snowballed from a simple three-page document I gave to my personal training clients. Those who followed my advice soon began to reap the rewards, and the feedback was excellent. Though I had believed it was a workable plan, I was still floored by the response. Everyone who tried it loved it. They passed it along to friends and family and before I knew it, people were asking me about my 'diet'. That's when I knew I had hit on something big.

The Lunch Box Diet was initially launched on the internet as an ebook, where it got rave reviews from top women's magazines. They were saying things like 'a way of life' and 'the best diet I've ever done' (*Elle* magazine, January 2008). I knew that the plan worked because I used it myself and my clients were telling me it worked for them, but it was an unbelievable feeling when top-rated women's publications were shouting it out to hundreds of thousands of people. That's what led us to where we are now – the printed book.

I don't want to be remembered for helping people to lose weight by drinking liquid diets and eating only one type of food, leaving them with no energy or zest for life. Instead, I want to help people to gain increased energy, improved concentration, better skin, no hunger pangs at work and improved overall health – the list goes on.

The great thing about the Lunch Box Diet is that after just a few days, you start to learn more about your body and it all happens quite naturally. If you are too strict about dieting or healthy eating, you will rebel. Of course, we all need an element of willpower to succeed but because you're reading this I assume you're ready to give it a go – so again, well done!

'I don't **want to be remembered** for helping people **to lose weight by** drinking liquid **diets and eating only one type of food**'

What Lies Ahead?

So what is this Lunch Box Diet? I'll go into depth later but as a very quick summary, the Lunch Box Diet is a fantastic, easy way of eating that lets you eat a normal breakfast and dinner and shows you how to 'graze' your way through the rest of the day. 'Grazing' means nibbling small quantities of food all day long, whenever you're hungry. The diet is based on some very simple principles, one of which you've known about since you were a child: eat your veggies. Don't run away! If you're not a vegetable lover, I'm going to teach you how easy it is to retrain your taste buds so that you will no longer want to hide your veggies in your napkin or feed them to the dog under the table.

I'll explain the low-down on healthy, effective, lasting weight loss. I'll guide you through the effect metabolism has on your ability to lose weight. I'll show you why you are far better off eating little and often than starving yourself. All those girls who starve themselves down to size 'negative-two' thin are asking for a heap of trouble in the future. At the very least, they'll simply gain the weight back (usually plus some) and find it more difficult to maintain an ideal body weight. In the worst case, they may end up with a serious, life-threatening eating disorder. I don't want that for you. I want you to be healthy and vibrant ... that's what sexy is.

Speaking of which, we're also going to look at the emotional aspects of eating. I've been in the personal training business long enough to know that issues surrounding weight gain go beyond what you put in your mouth. Sometimes it's a lot about why.

Once we're through all of the basics, I'm going to instruct you on how to follow the diet. I can't wait to show you all of its wonderful components and start you on the path to looking and feeling fabulous. I'll take you through the rainbow of vegetables and tell you all about the wonderful options when choosing lean protein (which go way beyond chicken). The Lunch Box Diet is easy to use if you don't eat meat, because you'll learn about other types of protein and how to incorporate them into your day.

'Don't run away! If you're not a vegetable lover, I'm going to teach you how easy it is to retrain your taste buds so that you will no longer want to hide your veggies'

I believe that 'sauce' should live up to its name by being 'saucy'. I'll show you how breaking up with those creamy dressings and heavy cheese sauces will be just as good for you as it was to dump that dreadful ex! Healthy sauce is anything but dull. My lunch boxes are delicious and yours will be too. I'll give you plenty of fabulous recipes to get you started.

Many diets today are based on reducing your carbohydrate intake. We'll talk about carbs and I'll show you why the low-carb craze is neither completely wrong nor completely right.

You'll be eating a normal breakfast and dinner in addition to the scrumptious contents of your lunch box – but what does 'normal' mean? I wish I could tell you that you can eat a monstrous stack of toast with bacon for breakfast and a 12-ounce T-bone steak, butter-stuffed baked potato and half a chocolate cake for dinner and still lose weight. Of course, I could say that – but then I'd be telling you a big fat lie! Don't worry. Conversely, I'm not going to tell you that all you can have is a carrot stick and a cup of hot water. What I will do is talk a bit about portions and provide you with some healthy ideas so we can gradually build you up to a healthier new you, forever!

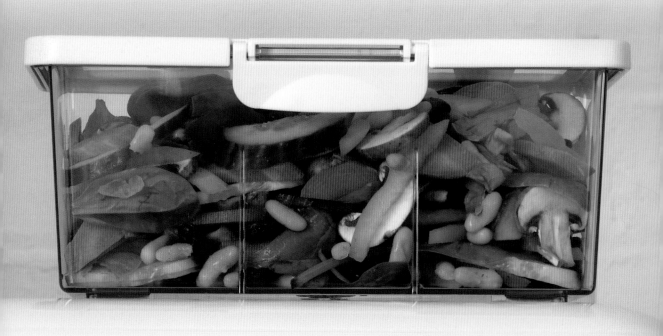

Unexpected Benefits

Don't you just love it when you get an unexpected bonus on your salary? You may have bought this book because you want to lose weight, but there's a hidden bonus because this diet goes way beyond weight loss. I didn't even realise how much so until I did some research. I'd simply chosen what I believed to be a healthy way of losing weight. When I looked into the food choices more deeply, I found out all sorts of things about what they can do in terms of your general health and I'm going to share that knowledge with you in chapter 8.

As well as getting a beautiful new body, your skin will improve and your hair will be healthier. Even more importantly, your heart will be healthier and you will be reducing your risk of developing disease. That's just a little bit of what goes on with your body when you eat the way I'm going to show you.

The best news of all is that you are going to feel better than you ever have in your life. You'll soon discover that this isn't merely a 'diet' – it's a revolutionary way of eating well that you will want to follow for life. Just give it seven days.

So, what are you waiting for? Welcome to your Lunch Box Diet.

You've tried and failed and tried and failed again. I'm sure you've blamed yourself

Chapter 2
Weight Loss: the Easy Way

I don't want to eat flavourless foods. I don't want to give up my favourites. I don't want to starve myself. I don't want to measure things or count calories or anything of the sort. And I'm sure you don't either.

Why? Because all of that is extremely stressful, as if life weren't stressful enough all on its own.

And guess what? All that stress could actually be making you heavier. We all react to stress differently. Since I began exercising, I tend to take out my frustrations in the gym. It wasn't always that way, though.

I used to let the pressures in my life affect me negatively. A long day in the office then a trip to the pub after work led to a sore head in the morning, followed by cravings for stodgy foods that would slow me down yet again, causing a snowball effect that left me with the movement and motivation of a sloth. Not a nice feeling.

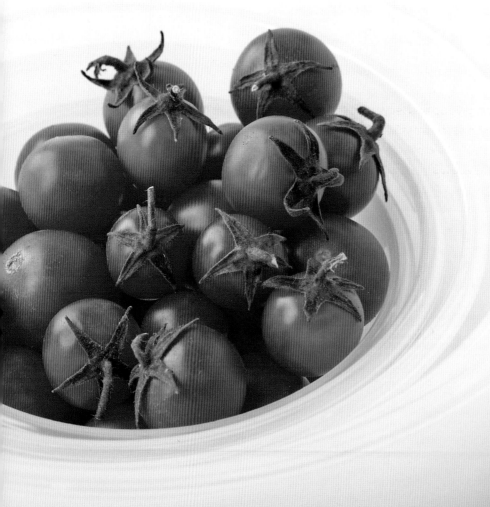

Mind and Body

We've heard for years about stress affecting our hearts. But it affects more, so much more. It affects nearly every part of our physical selves.

When we have very stressful lives, there are many physical symptoms. Joints ache, muscles feel weak, our hormones are out of whack, our immune systems are weakened, and these physical problems just add to the psychological pressure we're under. And guess what? As if the plate of brownies you consumed the other night after losing that promotion to your idiot colleague wasn't enough, the physical way in which your body responded to all that stress you've been under might have added a few extra pounds as well.

We produce the hormone cortisol when we are under stress and the kicker is that cortisol can cause you to produce more abdominal fat. Abdominal fat is undesirable aesthetically, and it also contains the most dangerous type of body fat. This is called 'visceral fat', and it has been linked to increased rates of cardiovascular disease and type II diabetes as well as breast cancer in women.

So, should you just give up and let yourself go? I mean, after all, it's not as if we can stop stressful things from happening, right? What do we do? First of all, you stop putting undue stress on yourself. Maybe it's inadvisable to tell the boss what you really think about his or her latest idiotic idea, but you can reduce personal stress by choosing not to follow ridiculously restrictive diets. Stop starving yourself or following plans that are clearly unhealthy. Stop denying yourself the foods you love. Stop eating flavourless foods because you've been told you'll lose weight if you follow a particular meal plan. It makes me so angry that people are adding to their life stresses because of their constant quest to be thin and perfect. It really doesn't need to be that way.

Simon's bite-sized tips

Reducing Stress

Learn a relaxation technique. Practising relaxation isn't difficult. All you need is five minutes in a quiet setting. Close your eyes, breathe in deeply through your nose and feel your belly fill up. Exhale through your nose feeling your belly empty. If thoughts come to mind, just let them go with the breath. Concentrate on the breath – that's it!

Listen to music. Keep music in the car, in the kitchen, in your bedroom, in the study, at the treadmill, in your gym bag ... everywhere! Choose the background music to your life. Music can relax us, it can fire us up, and it can touch on every emotion in between. It's also a great way of relieving stress.

Simon's bite-sized tips

Reducing Stress

Learn to let go of anger. Anger can help us if it produces the drive we need to overcome problems in our lives. However, when anger becomes resentment it only holds us back. Sometimes, we just have to let it go. Trust me, it takes a lot more energy to hold on to anger than it does to be happy. It's a choice you can make.

Free Yourself from Stress

I know you want to lose weight, but healthy weight loss doesn't have to be stressful. My clients are busy people who find that working out relieves stress from the daily grind. The last thing I want to do is add more stress to their lives. The Lunch Box Diet is convenient and versatile. People enjoy making and eating their own creations and coming up with new secret recipes. Colleagues, clients and friends are always trying to get a peek in my box, and I love to share ideas. If people didn't share then we would never learn.

Here's another piece of advice: 'Surround yourself with people you aspire to be like and you will end up being like them. Surround yourself with stressed people and you'll end up being stressed yourself.' The same can be said if you surround yourself with people who eat bad, junky foods. Have a think about who you are and how much of that is influenced by the people you surround yourself with. You may want to make a few changes in your life to help you on a more positive path, and this in turn will assist with your weight loss.

I've found that my clients like losing weight without the stress of traditional dieting. That's why I allow occasional indulgences while helping you to retrain your taste buds to enjoy healthy foods.

You'll find that when you eat a diet full of highly nutritious foods, you will be more energetic, stronger and healthier overall. When you are less susceptible to illness and feeling your best, stress is much easier to handle. In addition, you'll discover that there's no better stress-buster than a good session in the gym or other energetic pursuits. You don't have to exercise on the Lunch Box Diet but you'll probably be more inclined to get up and be active after only a short while on this diet.

Ultimately, my goal is to help you lose weight, learn to eat healthily for life, get you working out and do it all without stress. Leave those fad starvation diets behind and let's delve into a little science.

We tend to beat ourselves up for being overweight. We feel as though it's all about what we did or didn't do. Guess what? It's not all up to you. You weren't necessarily the one who failed. There's a better than zero chance that the diet failed you!

There are reasons why diets fail us. To understand this, you need to know a few basic nutritional principles. Don't worry, I'll make it fun! Keep reading.

The first is a simple maths equation.

weight maintenance:
what goes in = what goes out

What goes in is obviously the food you consume measured in calories, which is the measurement term used for energy. Your energy intake must be equivalent to what your body burns in order to simply maintain your weight. What doesn't get burned is stored as fat.

Burn, Baby, Burn

We burn energy day and night to perform the basic necessities of life: breathing, digestion, brain function and so forth. The amount of energy burned for these basic functions varies according to a person's size, age and sex. The larger the person, the harder the body has to work, so the more energy is burned. As we get older, we burn less energy – which may very well be why some of you bought this book in the first place. For the first time in your life, you might be experiencing weight gain.

Most of us do more during the day than simply breathing and digesting food (I hope!). How much more varies. Some of us have physically active jobs. Others spend the day sitting behind a desk. But we all have choices about what we do with our free time. For some, relaxing means lying on the sofa and for others it means going on a bracing hike.

Simon's bite-sized tips

Reducing Stress

Stop driving yourself crazy with guilt. Guilt is a wasted emotion. There are days when you get it all done and days when you don't. Accomplish the big things, the imperative things, but if you let a few little things slide to free up time for more important things like exercise or family time, that's okay!

I don't want you to count every calorie, nor to become a slave to the 'calories burned' function on your treadmill. However, you must adjust your eating to accommodate your activity level. It's just common sense.

Setting a Budget

Energy intake can be seen as a budget. When you wake up, you get a basic allowance according to your energy needs for the day that you can spend without paying the price of weight gain. All day long you spend this energy budget whenever you eat. If you take some form of exercise, you earn more energy so your budget for food is larger. You can eat more without gaining weight than others who are less active. We'll talk more about food budget and food choices when we get into the Lunch Box Diet itself, so grab a highlighter and mark up the page here.

For now, let's go back to our equation. I'm assuming you care less about weight maintenance and a lot more about weight loss. So, in looking at our equation, you can easily see that in order to lose weight, you need to do one of two things – or both.

Reduce what goes in (lower energy intake)

Increase what goes out (burn more energy)

Eat less and burn more energy (preferred)

Seems simple, right? For the most part, it is. But how much should you cut out of your diet in order to lose weight at an optimum rate? Again I don't want you to count but for the sake of understanding, I'll tell you a bit more. One pound of body weight is more or less equivalent to 3,500 calories. Rather convenient considering there are seven days in a week. You can quickly see that if you reduce your energy intake by 500 calories a day or burn an additional 500 calories (about a 40-minute jog/run on the treadmill), you should theoretically lose about a pound a week.

You might be tempted to adjust this even more severely to lose weight more quickly. The fact is, in order to lose weight effectively – in other words keep the weight off – slow and steady is the key. There are guidelines to what people say is safe, but we need to remember that, depending on your current weight and the changes to your diet and exercise, weight will drop off at different rates per individual – usually the heavier you are the more initially and then less as your weight comes down closer to maintenance level. What we want to steer away from is a ridiculous calorie chop where you're taking in a stupidly low amount of calories per day, but don't worry, that's not going to happen here! You won't be able to continue a very low-calorie diet forever and once you resume eating more than carrot sticks and hot water, you'll gain it back. It also mucks up your metabolism, which we'll discuss later (see page 25). Fortunately with the Lunch Box Diet, it's a sustainable plan that you can see working long term as part of your new, happy lifestyle!

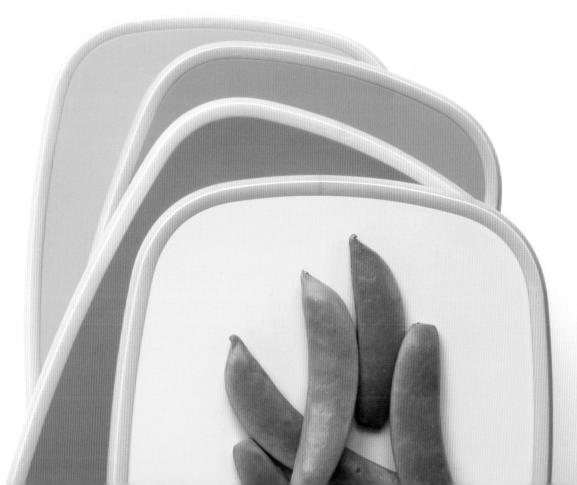

Why Diets Fail

The majority of fad diets are nothing more than very low-calorie diets with a gimmick or smoke screen to cover up this fact. Whether you're told to eat a grapefruit or drink a strange mixture, at the end of the day, you've consumed fewer calories, often to the extreme.

At best, there's a small grain of truth in each theory but only to a minuscule degree. All that these diets do is, once again, cover up the fact that calories are being restricted, no matter what horse and pony show went into making you not eat. And most of the time, you will not be able to stick with it because people, quite simply, get hungry! We like to eat. We don't usually enjoy hunger pangs, weakness and dizziness. We do enjoy treats like chocolate and crisps. We can go some time without these things but if you ignore a craving long enough, chances are it'll come back to bite you on the bum and a little craving for a taste of chocolate will snowball into eating an entire box!

Let's recap:

- **Healthy weight loss relies on one equation.**
- **Fad diets fail because most are very low-calorie diets (VLCDs for short).**
- **Fad diets fail because they are too stringent.**
- **Fad diets fail because they are not built for the long run.**

Fad diets fail because starving yourself will mess with your metabolism! Metabolism? I know what you're thinking: 'You said you'd keep it simple!' I will, I will.

The Bear Necessities

Metabolism is the rate at which our bodies burn calories or, in other words, fuel. The higher the metabolism, the faster the fuel is burned. The lower the metabolism, the slower fuel is burned. When you starve yourself, you end up lowering your metabolism.

The best way I can explain how metabolism aids in weight loss is to talk about bears. Huh? You heard me right. A bear spends all summer fattening itself up. It has to fatten up to get through the whole winter without eating. A bear's metabolism slows way, way down during hibernation. This is the body's way of preserving all that fat the bear put on last summer. Good for the bear, not so good for you. When was the last time you saw a bear having to wear a backless cocktail dress?

When we starve ourselves, we do the same thing to our metabolism as hibernation does to the bear's metabolism. Without any new fuel source, your body works as efficiently as possible by lowering its metabolism to conserve any existing fuel. It stores what it can. Conversely, when you eat small amounts of food frequently throughout the day (graze) rather than starve yourself, your metabolism remains at optimum fuel-burning level. It can rely on getting fuel every one to two hours and therefore it burns fuel instead of storing it.

That being said, you can't eat high-calorie, high-fat food every one to two hours and still lose weight. So, what do you eat? That's where my diet plan comes into play.

In designing the diet, I knew I wanted my clients to graze but I didn't want to give them a blanket instruction to eat all day. They needed to eat foods that had a lot of nutritional punch per bite without a lot of calories. They needed something lasting and tasty yet without a ton of calories. Some foods are just fattening and may be low in nutrients. Those are the types of foods that, when consumed regularly, make us fat.

'When you eat small amounts of food frequently throughout the day (graze) rather than starve yourself, your metabolism remains at optimum fuel-burning level'

Beyond the Mirror

In a world where thin is in and obesity is (what the heck rhymes with obesity?) not, it's tough to be heavy for a whole plethora of reasons. Many of you are reading this book because you're tired of being heavy and have chosen to do something about it. Good on you!

I've seen so many people literally change their entire lives when they drop the pounds. For most people, food means so much more than just fuel for our bodies. We use it at nearly every celebration: birthday cake, Easter eggs, and don't even get me started on the days of feasting around Christmas. We're taught at a very, very young age that sweets and cake are pleasant and that pleasant things make us feel good. If you scrape a knee, you get a plaster followed by a lolly to turn off the tears.

The lolly doesn't fix the wound, but distracts the child's attention from the pain. When you're sad, lonely, restless, anxious or angry, your 'lolly' might be chocolate cake or a fast-food burger that distracts you from your emotions. For a brief moment, you're preoccupying yourself by doing something pleasurable. Unfortunately, it's not lasting and, just like the lolly, it doesn't fix the wound. Food can't fix what's really wrong.

What's worse is that the excess food is only complicating your life further. It's a vicious cycle. We eat too much because we're depressed, we gain weight, we get more depressed, we eat more, we gain more and so on. Stop the cycle! When you start treating your body right, when you take control of your weight instead of letting it control you, you empower yourself to make other changes in your life.

You may not be able to fix everything overnight but a journey begins with a single step. You have taken that step by purchasing this book and trusting me. I won't let you down! I'll be with you on that journey.

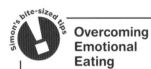

Simon's bite-sized tips

Overcoming Emotional Eating

Next time you overeat or indulge in fattening comfort foods, write down the emotions you are feeling.

When you feel the urge to eat, ask yourself, 'Am I physically hungry or emotionally hungry?'

Keep temptation out of the fridge and cupboards. If instant gratification isn't available, you're less likely to eat for the wrong reasons.

Go for a walk, run or hit the gym the next time you're angry, sad or anxious.

Before you reach for that pizza slice, stop, close your eyes and visualize the life you want for yourself. Will the pizza slice get you there? Will it fix what's wrong?

For starters I urge everyone to join the Lunch Box Diet community (see page 224) at www.lunchboxdiet.co.uk – go and do it now. I will send you regular emails to keep you motivated and this is key to your success! I'm constantly coming up with new techniques, tips and tricks and I'll share these with you. How about that for an added bonus?

Though looking good will be a big part of the end result of following this diet plan, what's most important is how you will perceive yourself from the inside out once you begin the Lunch Box Diet. Eating healthily means feeling good. More energy, less illness, less chance of developing diseases related to obesity. You'll be able to enjoy your life.

Whenever you're feeling down, remember this word:

> ## BELIEVE!
>
> Believe in this diet.
> **Believe in your efforts.**
> Believe in me.
> **Believe, above all,**
> **in you and your abilities!**
>
> **We'll get there! I promise!**

Okay, enough pep talk. Can you feel the energy? If not, put the book down for a minute, get off your bum and jog around the couch ten times.

Ready? Let's get to work. Turn the page.

Simon's bite-sized tips

Kids and Emotional Eating

I really want what's best for you and your kiddos. I hope these little tips will get you thinking about what you can do.

Try not to use food as a comfort with your kids. Instead of a lolly when they scrape their knee, how about a hug or kiss after the plaster? Perhaps suggest a trip to the book shop.

Dump the idea of 'finish your food'. Don't say things like 'If you don't finish your food, you can't have dessert.' Try to trust what they tell you about their bodies.

Don't make food a focal point. Get your kids moving more by planning fun activities such as hikes, bike rides, or some other type of family adventure.

Slowly replace any fattening foods kept in the house with healthier alternatives.

Suggest a trip to the park after dinner instead of serving dessert.

You made it! We finally get to delve into this life-changing eating plan. You're days away from feeling fantastic!

Chapter 3

The Lunch Box Diet

Hard to believe? Believe it, because in just seven days you're going to feel the effects of optimum nutrition. Work independently for a month, following the lunch box system, or finish my 28-day plan and you'll be on top of the world.

The Box

Okay, remember our little chat about healthy weight loss, grazing and metabolism (see page 25)? You're now going to find out why you had to go back to school for a bit.

Here's what you will be doing:

1. **Eat a healthy breakfast (or your normal breakfast and build up to a healthier one).**
2. **Graze from your lunch box between breakfast and dinner.**
3. **Eat a healthy dinner (or your normal dinner and build up to a healthier one).**

The lunch box concept is simply the most effective and easiest way to control most people's nutrition because:

- You know exactly what you're eating.
- You don't have to plan and prepare meal after meal.
- You will have a choice of foods that will enable you to enjoy eating from your plastic friend!

Lunch boxes are quick to put together, tasty and will give you bucketloads of energy! Not to mention the added health benefits that we'll discuss later in Chapter 8.

When working with personal training clients, I always ask them to keep a record of their food intake (a food diary) for about a week to get an idea of what they like and how they eat. I often find that the pitfalls of their dieting behaviour have a lot to do with their busy lifestyles. I suggest you keep a food diary yourself and note down your own thoughts on your food consumption; you may get a bit of a shock, but that's fine. Just write down everything you eat for a week, including any drinks, and the times you eat, plus the exercise you take.

Finding healthy options during a normal, busy day is extremely difficult. My clients would either go without because they didn't have good choices, or they would opt for the fast-food or vending-machine items out of sheer necessity. We simply don't make informed choices when we're hungry, and that's why the Lunch Box Diet is such a good way of eating. By grazing out of a box that you prepare ahead of time, you will be eliminating two major barriers to healthy weight loss.

• You won't end up choosing junk because your blood sugar levels will be more balanced.
• You won't devour the contents of the fridge as soon as you get a chance.

I'll talk about breakfast and dinner in a bit (see chapter 6) but for now, let's concentrate on the box itself.

The Method

Remember: I don't want you to have the hassle of measuring and weighing and counting calories. That's why I keep it simple. If you can count, you can do this!

You'll need a container with a lid that has a volume of between 2 and 5 litres. To find the volume of your box, simply pour water into it from a measuring jug. Mine is about the size of a shoebox and I'd class myself as an average-sized male. The size will become more apparent to you as you go along with the diet and adjustments can easily be made. The simple rule here is to pack more than you think you'll need at first and then drop the box size (or simply the amount of food you put in it) once you're used to the system. The main thing is not to pack too little and go hungry.

The idea is that you will eat a few mouthfuls from your box every hour or so – never to the point that you're full, only until you're satisfied. This is what grazing is. Your brain takes around 20 to 30 minutes to catch up with your stomach so take a few bites and if in 20 to 30 minutes you're still hungry, take a few more bites. Yep, it's as easy as that.

You'll learn quickly that you can be easily satisfied on less when you graze because you're constantly refuelling the body. Your stomach will adjust to less food just as it does the opposite when we overeat. When you pig out at a meal you stretch the stomach, making it more difficult to feel satisfied at the next meal, and you're left on the sofa feeling tired and bloated. Yep, it's that vicious cycle again, which you will now break!

Grazing does the exact opposite, super-fast, leaving you brimming with energy. What this means is that over time, you can reduce the size of your lunch box as you'll need less to feel satisfied. I never want you to feel hungry – that's the main thing; but if you are regularly having trouble finishing your box, just cut down the contents. It's as easy as that!

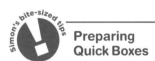

Simon's bite-sized tips

Preparing Quick Boxes

Pick pre-cooked meats and mixed vegetable packs.

Cook extra meat at your evening meal to put in your box the next day.

Stock up on herbs and other dressing ingredients from Group C.

Buy frozen vegetables.

Bribe your partner to make your box at the same time as they're making their own.

What Do You Put in the Box?

There are three groups that you will be choosing from:

Group A: Vegetables – 45–60 per cent of your box by volume

Group B: Lean Protein – 15–30 per cent of your box by volume

Group C: Sauce – 10 per cent of your box by volume

And as an optional extra ONLY if you have high activity levels or diabetes:

Group D: Active Carbs System – 0–30 per cent quantity depends on energy requirements

As you can see, your largest portion of the box is comprised of vegetables. You'll be choosing five veggies from the Group A list. The key here is to be colourful. You're most likely to create the perfect combination of nutrients when you choose a rainbow of vegetables because different colours indicate that they contain different kinds of the nutrients known as phytochemicals.

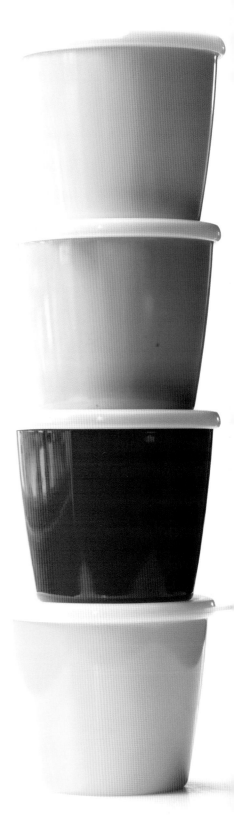

Group A: Vegetables
45–60% Pick 5

Red

Beetroots
Peppers
Radishes
Rhubarb
Tomatoes (yeah, its fruit)
Watermelon (ditto)

Orange & yellow

Carrots
Pumpkins
Squash
Sweetcorn
Sweet potatoes

Green

Artichokes
Asparagus
Avocados
Broccoli
Brussels sprouts
Celery

Cucumber
Green beans
Green leaves
Mangetout
Peas
Sugarsnap peas

'Blue' (white)

Cauliflower
Leeks
Mushrooms
Parsnips
Shallots and onions

Indigo & violet

Aubergines
Cabbage
Turnips

Whenever you can, use fresh, raw, organic vegetables. For the ones that need to be cooked, you can steam, grill, oven bake or microwave them. Please don't torture your veggies by boiling the life and the nutrients out of them and don't add oil or butter when preparing them. You'll be adding flavour to your box later, so be patient!

Now, you might be thinking 'I'm not a rabbit, Simon! I can't possibly eat all those weeds and things!' No worries! If your taste buds are used to greasy, calorie-laden foods like pizza, bacon and eggs, cakes and sweets, you'll have a bit of adjustment to make. All that sugar, sodium and saturated fat does indeed taste good but what's the price? Your belly, bum and thighs. Not to mention clogged arteries, diabetes, high blood pressure, bad skin and hair ... the list goes on and on.

Individual tastes vary from person to person, partly due to our genetic make-up and partly because of the tastes we are introduced to as very young children. Some people might be under-tasters and some may be super-tasters. This has to do with the number of taste buds per square centimetre on your tongue. Under-tasters with fewer taste buds tend to pile on the sugar and go heavy with salt. Vegetables taste bland for these folks. On the other hand, super-tasters with a lot of taste buds might find some veggies overwhelmingly bitter.

It's not hard to retrain your taste buds and get to know your vegetables (check out my bite-sized tips). Truth is, if you don't, I can safely say you'll continue to have weight issues and be unhealthy as well. Fact of the matter is, we weren't put on this earth to eat crisps and chocolate bars. Ask yourself, did Mother Nature grow it that way? We were provided with certain basic foods that are good for us in their natural state. By eating naturally, we're giving ourselves what we need. If you don't like vegetables it's because you've been eating rubbish for so long that you've got used to it. But if you want to be vibrant, sexy, full of energy and taut around the stomach then you will need to acquire a taste for vegetables at some point.

Simon's bite-sized tips

Vegetable Tastebud Builder

I encourage you to use the guide below to wean your way to liking vegetables – your key to a healthier lifestyle. Pick the option that applies to you.

You love vegetables so much that you could have been one in your previous life.

Fantastic! You can use the Lunch Box Diet up to seven days a week if you wish.

You're a fan of vegetables, but like to be naughty sometimes.

No problem. Use the diet in your working week and take a couple of days off at weekends to reward yourself.

I don't mind vegetables but I prefer other foods.

Okay, so bring the diet into your life three days a week and increase that once you begin to feel the benefits.

Vegetables? Sure! I love ketchup and lettuce on my burger!

You should have a lunch box once a week to begin with and try adding another day every couple of weeks to gradually educate your digestive system and taste buds.

Group B: Protein
15–30% Pick 1

Here's where you'll be getting your staying power. Protein takes longer to digest than carbohydrates and therefore leaves you feeling satisfied longer. Pick one type of protein source for each lunch box.

Choose quality meat and avoid the pre-packaged stuff that is mostly fillers and water and is poor in nutritional value. Although better-quality meats cost a bit more, you'll quickly realise that you need less of them to satisfy you. I also advocate buying organic if you can afford it (see page 80 for the reasons why) but it's not imperative.

Beef

Lean cuts: sirloin, rump steak, topside, silverside

Lamb

Shoulder, rack or cutlets

Fish

Oily fish: salmon, sardines, herring, mackerel, trout, tuna
White fish: sole, haddock, cod, sea bass, sea bream, skate

Shellfish

Prawns, shrimp, crab, lobster, mussels, cockles, scallops, oysters

Poultry

White meat: chicken or turkey breast

Pork

Pork and lean cuts of ham

Dairy

Eggs

Plant sources

Tofu, chickpeas, beans, seeds and nuts

Simon's bite-sized tips

Money Saving

Proteins can be pricy, so here are the ones with the best nutritional bang for your buck:

Eggs

Beans (aduki, blackeye, borlotti, flageolet, haricot, red kidney)

Chickpeas

Lentils

Tinned fish (sardines, pilchards, mackerel, salmon, tuna)

Turkey breast

Group C: Dressing
10%

Sprinkle a dressing into your box after adding vegetables and protein, to bring it alive. I like hot sauces, herbs and black pepper – make your own or buy them (see page 91), but read the labels for added sugar and E numbers. Don't worry about the calories since you're only sprinkling or drizzling.

Cheese (lightly sprinkled – all types)
Chinese-style dressings (made with tahini, rice vinegar, sesame oil and soy sauce)
Chutney (see page 214 for recipe)
Fruit, chopped (apple, watermelon, pear, strawberries)
Garlic, ginger and onion
Guacamole (avocado, tomato, lime juice, red onion, chilli)
Harissa paste (made with chilli, garlic, caraway, coriander and olive oil)
Herbs (fresh – any kind at all)
Hummus (mashed chickpeas, tahini, lemon juice and garlic)
Lemon, lime, apple or orange juice
Marinades (see page 212 for recipes)
Oils (olive or nut – just a splash)
Olives and capers
Pepper sauce (my favourite!)
Pesto (see page 215 for recipe)
Salsa (see page 214 for recipe)
Sauerkraut
Soy sauce (choose the 'light' varieties)
Tapenade (olive paste with lemon juice and garlic)
Teriyaki sauce (see page 213 for recipe)
Thai fish sauce (made with anchovies)
Tomato sauce (fresh, see page 87 for recipe)
Tzatziki (fresh, see page 214 for recipe)
Vinegar (plain, fruit-flavoured, cider or wine, or vinaigrettes)
Wasabi, soy and ginger (traditional sushi accompaniments)

Once again, be creative. I've provided you with some suggestions and you can invent your own combinations.

A little oil goes a long way. Though olive oil and walnut oil are good fats, they have a strong flavour and you shouldn't drench your lunch box in them. You can always add a bit more if you need to, but don't forget that your veggies and meats will be absorbing the flavouring as they marinate in the box throughout the day, making the taste more intense. You don't want everything to taste like pickles by 5pm! You might consider tossing in a small, sealed container of sauce so that you can add extra later if you need to.

Group D: Active Carbs

Extra 0–30%

Depending on the kind of lifestyle you lead, you may require a little more energy in your box to keep you going. If you sit in an office most of the day, I'd like you to stick with the standard box with groups A, B and C, and see how your energy levels compare to normal. Chances are if you're used to eating three times a day you will notice a significant improvement as your blood sugar levels stabilise. You'll be surprised how much energy you get just by picking at your box.

I never want you to lack energy, so if you feel sluggish, add in one active carb from the list below and see how you perform. Bear in mind that there could be other factors affecting your energy level, such as lack of sleep. You should also add an active carb if you suffer from diabetes.

Barley	Rye bread or crackers
Brown or wild rice	Whole pieces of fruit
Buckwheat, bulgur wheat	Wholegrain bread
Oatcakes	Wholegrain couscous
Quinoa	Wholewheat pasta

If you are taking an exercise class or going to the gym, leave around an hour and a half for your food to digest beforehand. Take your box with you so you can replenish your energy directly after your session instead of grabbing unhealthy snacks. Alternatively, a banana is a good post-gym snack.

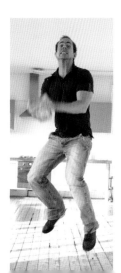
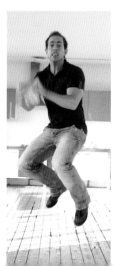
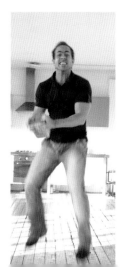
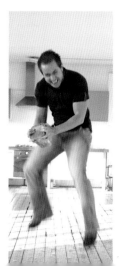

Let's just recap the box contents

- **Group A: Vegetables** – Grab a selection of five and throw them into your box.
- **Group B: Protein** – Choose one protein source per box.
- **Group C: Dressing** – Essential to add flavour; a little goes a long way.
- **Group D: Active carbs** – Only add these if you have high activity levels.

The Lunch Box Diet Tremor

You've prepared your box for the day and it's already looking pretty tasty, but how do you get it bursting with flavour? It's time for a box tremor! Seal your lid, grasp the edges for extra seal protection and perform the 5-second tremor. Go. You'll be surprised at how much difference this makes to the flavour of your box. Those tomatoes will split, seeping their juices; beetroots will blast their purple flavour around; and those herbs and spices will trickle onto every leaf. Yummy!

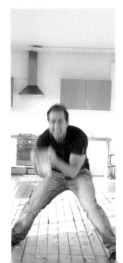 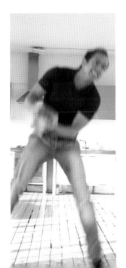 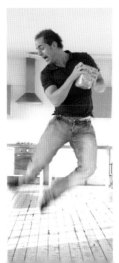 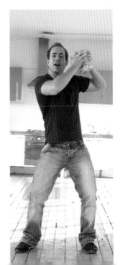

Choosing a great combination of colours and flavours adds aesthetic appeal and provides optimum nutrition

Chapter 4

Your Rainbow of Great Flavours

Group A: Vegetables

Eating lots of vegetables is a great way to achieve healthy weight loss because they are low in calories and very versatile. If you grew up on tinned green beans and corn, then you might not be aware of all the different choices.

Raw vs Cooked

When vegetables are raw, they contain all the goodness that Mother Nature intended. On the whole, when we start manipulating them in the kitchen, little by little they lose nutritional value. Have you ever looked at the water in a pan in which you've boiled broccoli? It's green, right? Carrot water is orange. Magic trick? No. What you're looking at is the phytochemicals that you've just boiled out of the vegetable.

Phytochemicals give vegetables their bright beautiful colours and they also provide you with powerful substances called antioxidants. Our bodies are full of little guys called free radicals that are created by environmental factors such as sunlight and pollution and other things that we ingest. They create quite a bit of damage, ageing cells and damaging tissues. Antioxidants have the ability to neutralise free radicals and rid the body of them, thus helping to prevent cellular and tissue damage and protect you from life-threatening diseases such as cancer. Which is a good reason to eat as many as you can.

Another reason to avoid too much unnecessary cooking is that it breaks down the fibre content of vegetables and makes it less effective. Fibre is the indigestible portion of plants that is necessary for a healthy digestive system. It helps move the stomach contents through the digestive system and aids in elimination. In other words, it stops you getting constipated.

Vegetables that need to be cooked can be lightly steamed, microwaved, briefly roasted in a hot oven or grilled. Be careful what you add to them, though. Butter, cheese, dressings and other types of heavy sauce are popular ways of preparing vegetables but try vinegars, pepper sauces, black pepper, onion, shallots or garlic instead to avoid adding fat and calories to such wonderful little packages of nutrition.

Red

Beetroots

The 'sweet beet' is finally gaining the recognition it deserves. Beetroots are packed full of nutrients such as folic acid, vitamin C and potassium and they contain fibre and other antioxidants as well.

Selection: Though we most often think of beetroots as 'red' they can actually be orange or white in colour and their size can range from little golf balls to baseballs. When purchased with their greens still attached, make sure the leaves are fresh-looking and not wilted. Without the leaves, beets should be of good colour and heavy, devoid of wrinkly or sprouting skin.

Preparation: They are incredibly versatile in the kitchen and can be prepared in a number of ways. Peel them and cut into chunks then either place them in a quarter cup of water in a microwavable dish and cook on high for around 10 minutes or steam them on the stove until tender. Don't boil the nutrients out of them the way grandma used to do. Quite excellent served cold, they are perfect for your lunch box! And don't forget to save their greens and roots – these are edible and full of nutrients. Just wash and toss in your lunch box.

Simon's bite-sized tips

Folic Acid

Folic acid (or folate) is extremely important for pregnant women, as it helps prevent the birth defect spina bifida. It is also important for heart health and mental health, as low folate has been linked to depression.

Peppers

We'll discuss the spicy, hot guys on page 86, but here I'm talking about bell peppers, which can be red, yellow, orange or green. They add flavour and zest but have very few calories and a lot of antioxidants. (Remember those things we talked about that neutralise free radicals, so are anti-ageing and anti-cancer?) Red peppers contain more than three times as much vitamin C as oranges as well as being a good supply of beta-carotene (which the body converts to vitamin A). In addition, they contain a fair amount of fibre and vitamin B6.

Selection: The colour should be vibrant and rich. Stay away from pale peppers as they are of poorer quality and nutritional value. They should be heavy and firm with no soft spots.

Preparation: Wash, cut a circle around the stem and pull out the core. Rinse the seeds out. With a sharp knife, cut in half and slice into strips then remove the remaining white membrane where the core was attached. Leave in strips or chop them up. Your choice!

Radishes

Radishes are great for flavour, colour and vitamin C as well as an antioxidant called indole (see left). Though we tend to think of 'red' radishes, there are other varieties and their flavour changes from the sweet white icicles to the sharp black radish.

Selection: Choose healthy-looking radishes with bright, fresh greens.

Preparation: Chop off the greens before storing and they will last longer in the fridge. When ready to use, simply rinse and chop to desired size.

Simon's bite-sized tips

Indole

The antioxidant indole has been shown to block the effects of excess oestrogen in the body, which leads some scientists to believe that it may reduce the chances of developing breast cancer. Good levels of indole can be found in the brassica group of vegetables, including broccoli, cabbage, cauliflower and sprouts.

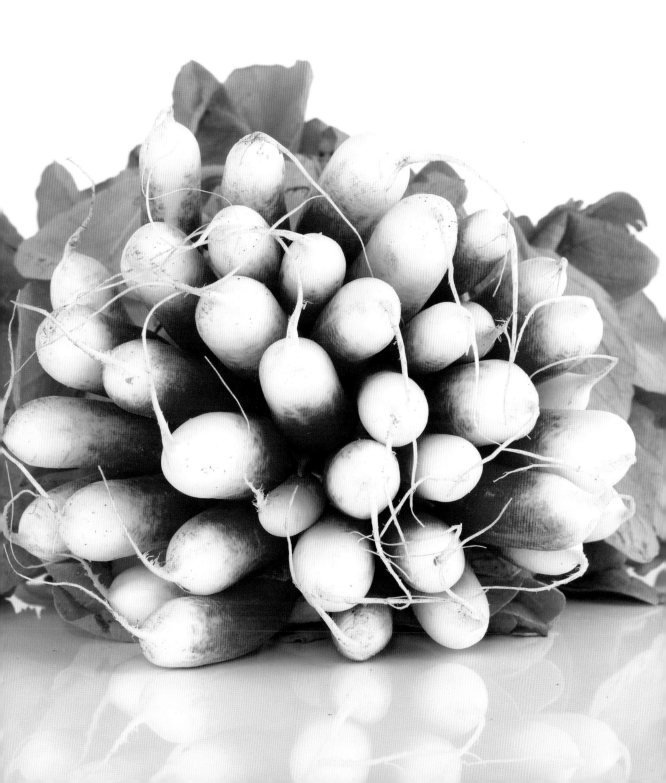

Rhubarb

Rhubarb's tart flavour makes it a great addition to your lunch box; however, the traditional method of cooking rhubarb with tons of sugar needs to be modified. Rhubarb offers fibre, potassium and calcium and 100 grams of rhubarb (without sugar) is only 7 calories!

Selection: Rhubarb should be crisp and glossy. The colour can range from pale green or pink all the way to a deep red colour and doesn't matter when you're making a selection. The most tender stalks will be less than 3cm thick. Remove any traces of leaves as they contain a corrosive toxin called oxalic acid.

Preparation: Rhubarb is too tart to eat alone but it need not be drenched in sugar. Use sweet berries or sweet cider vinegar in the water when you boil it, with maybe just a teaspoonful of honey to taste.

Tomatoes

Tomatoes are a universal favourite used widely in many different cuisines. They're full of antioxidants, including the super-antioxidant lycopene, which has strong anti-cancer properties and has been shown to reduce the harmful process of oxidation of LDL ('bad') cholesterol in the blood. Try heirloom tomatoes if you can find them. They are as varied in flavour as they are in shape and colour. These charismatic guys can be green, yellow, red, orange and even a deep colour that looks almost black. Red and orange are the sweetest and green is tart. Try sun-blush and sundried tomatoes as well for a more intense flavour.

Selection: Steer clear of hot-house tomatoes. These pale guys contain up to 50 per cent fewer phytochemicals than they would have had if they'd been grown in the sun and left on the vine to ripen. If a tomato isn't a gorgeous red, it probably isn't very good. Choose tomatoes that are firm but not rock hard and let them sit out on the counter in an attractive dish.

They are ripe when they feel supple yet not too soft. Store tomatoes in a cool place on the countertop. You can speed up the ripening process by placing them in a brown paper bag.

Preparation: Tomatoes are wonderful chopped up, used for fresh salsa (see page 214) or roasted, and go wonderfully with nearly any lunch box combination.

Watermelon

A fruit, but worthy of a veggie listing and great in your lunch-box because of its sweet, mouth-watering flavour and its beta-carotene, lycopene and potassium content.

Selection: Watermelon is definitely seasonal and, as a rule of thumb, the less expensive, the better the fruit. Produce that is in abundance is generally the freshest and markets put them on sale because of this reason. Choose seedless varieties for convenience and make sure it is firm and has no soft spots. Look for a lighter-coloured rough patch somewhere that indicates that the fruit has had some ripening time lying on the ground in the field.

Preparation: I like to chop it up and sprinkle it in a 'salty' lunch box combination to take the edge off the salt. See the 'Trim Turkey' lunch box recipe on page 198.

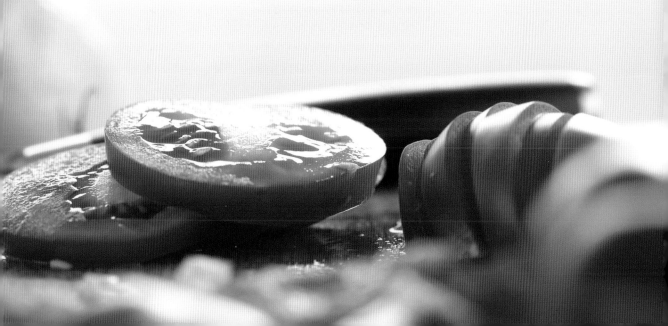

Orange & Yellow

Carrots

Can't forget the good old carrot. Full of beta-carotene, this endearing veggie is probably the easiest to snack on. Ever seen a rabbit wearing glasses? Seriously, it's long been known that the beta-carotene found in carrots is great for eye health. They are an easy way to add orange to your lunch box and should be a staple in your fridge.

Selection: Crisp and fresh-looking is the key, with nice bright orange colouring.

Preparation: Most of us are pretty familiar with carrots, so the only piece of advice I have to add is that the pre-washed organic baby carrots sold in the bag are a nice convenience to have on hand for those rushed mornings.

Pumpkin

Many relate pumpkins to autumn décor, but the smaller-variety pumpkins can be cooked and eaten. They are loaded with alpha-carotene and low in calories. They add a delicious sweet touch to your lunch box and can be substituted in other dishes where you might use winter squash or sweet potato.

Selection: Choose the small, sweet varieties that are becoming more and more popular as pumpkin is touted by gourmet chefs as a culinary delight. Look for ones that are heavy for their size, devoid of blemishes or soft spots, and have at least 2cm of stem. Off season, tinned pumpkin can be substituted but make sure you don't purchase the sweetened, seasoned type intended for pumpkin pie.

Preparation: To prepare a fresh pumpkin, you need to rinse it, cut a hole in the top and scrape out the seeds and stringy stuff. Pumpkins can be baked in the oven with their skin on (word to the wise: line your baking tin with parchment paper so the sticky juice doesn't ruin it) or you can peel the skin, cut into cubes and steam or microwave. To use tinned pumpkin, just open the tin and scoop out.

Squash

You may be tempted not to cut into these beauties and just leave them out for a centrepiece, but slice away because they contain tons of nutrients including beta-carotene, vitamin C, niacin, phosphorus and potassium. There are many varieties, such as acorn, blue hubbard, buttercup, butternut, spaghetti squash and many, many more. The flavours and textures range from squash to squash, so experiment! Some are great by themselves and others are better suited for complementing dishes.

Selection: Make sure they are heavy for their size and devoid of soft spots.

Preparation: For lunch box purposes, I recommend roasting. Simply slice the squash in half, remove the seeds and cut away the rind. Cut the flesh into cubes and season to taste. Roast in a hot oven until they are lightly browned (about 20 minutes).

Alternatively, you can bake it in the oven in its peel and remove the rind afterwards. This will give it the consistency of mashed potatoes.

Sweetcorn

Sweetcorn contains vitamin C, fibre and B complex vitamins. B vitamins regulate a whole plethora of cellular functions in the body. They are important for the kidneys, the heart and blood vessels and the metabolism. Sweetcorn is incredibly versatile and can be eaten alone, sprinkled over salads, and added to salsas. Buy it ripe in season or look for organic frozen sweetcorn. Tinned corn has a lower vitamin content. Make sure it has no added salt or sugar.

Frozen Sweetcorn

Frozen organic sweetcorn is perfectly acceptable; just microwave for a minute before tossing in your box.

Selection: If you are buying corn in its husk, peel it first. It's a real bummer to get home, peel back an ear and find rotten corn on half of the cob.

Preparation: Don't overcook this wonderful treat! Boil the cob until you can pierce a kernel with a fork and it sort of 'pops'. Eat it like that or scrape it into your lunch box or salsa.

Sweet Potatoes

Sweet potatoes are packed full of nutrients and well worth the calories. They contain beta-carotene (the orange flesh has the most) and other antioxidants, as well as fibre. Beta-carotene is needed for vitamin A production in the body, which is involved in white blood cell production and thus affects your immunity to disease. It also plays an important role in bone health. Sweet potatoes are one of the higher-calorie items in the vegetable component of the Lunch Box Diet but you only need small portions.

Selection

Sweet potatoes are often confused with yams, which are a large root vegetable indigenous to Asia and Africa. Orange-fleshed sweet potatoes (moist) are usually called yams while the drier (yellow/white flesh) variety are labelled sweet potatoes. The orange variety are far more flavoursome as well as more nutritious.

Preparation

Sweet potatoes can be baked for dinner just as you would bake a potato or cubed and steamed to be thrown into your lunch box. If baking for dinner, don't muck it up with a ton of butter. Instead, opt for a dollop of low-fat plain yoghurt with a bit of pepper and sea salt sprinkled on top after baking. Delicious!

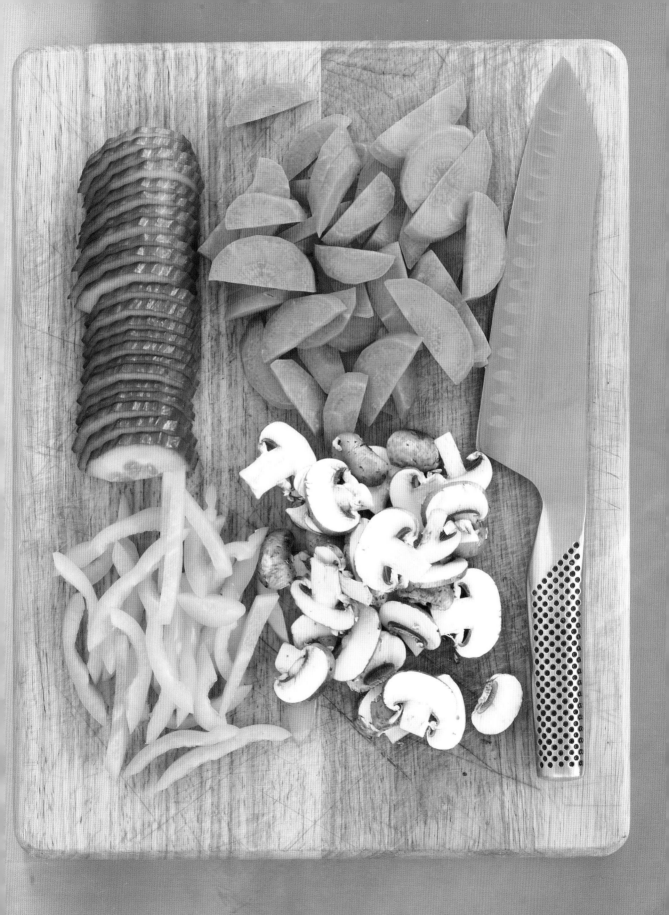

Green

Artichokes

Artichokes are a source of magnesium, copper and folic acid as well as other B vitamins, vitamin K and calcium. Extracts of artichokes have been found to have a protective effect on liver cells. It's also been found to reduce cholesterol. High in fibre and containing protein, these guys are just as good for you as they are delicious.

Selection: Jerusalem artichokes are root vegetables. I'm talking about globe artichokes here, with lots of leaves packed around the heart. Look for nice, tight leaves and density.

Preparation: Artichokes are well worth the work. Steam them then pull off the leaves one by one and scrape the fleshy side of the leaf with your teeth. Traditionally, leaves are dipped in melted butter but you could substitute more healthy sauces, such as garlic/olive oil/herb combinations. For your lunch box, I recommend marinating the steamed artichoke heart in vinegar, herbs and a bit of olive oil. Tinned artichoke hearts have less nutritional value than fresh but are still worthwhile.

Asparagus

Asparagus tips are delicious and truly a delectable, tender delight when in season but can be tough and woody at other times. Asparagus contains a lot of folic acid and beta-carotine and the powerful antioxidant glutathinone as well as vitamin C.

Selection: Asparagus is usually an early summer vegetable. It over-ripens quickly and, if not properly transported, it can look rather limp. Make sure the asparagus you pick is firm.

Preparation: Break off any woody ends. Asparagus is wonderful lightly steamed and drizzled with freshly squeezed lemon and a smidgeon of olive oil.

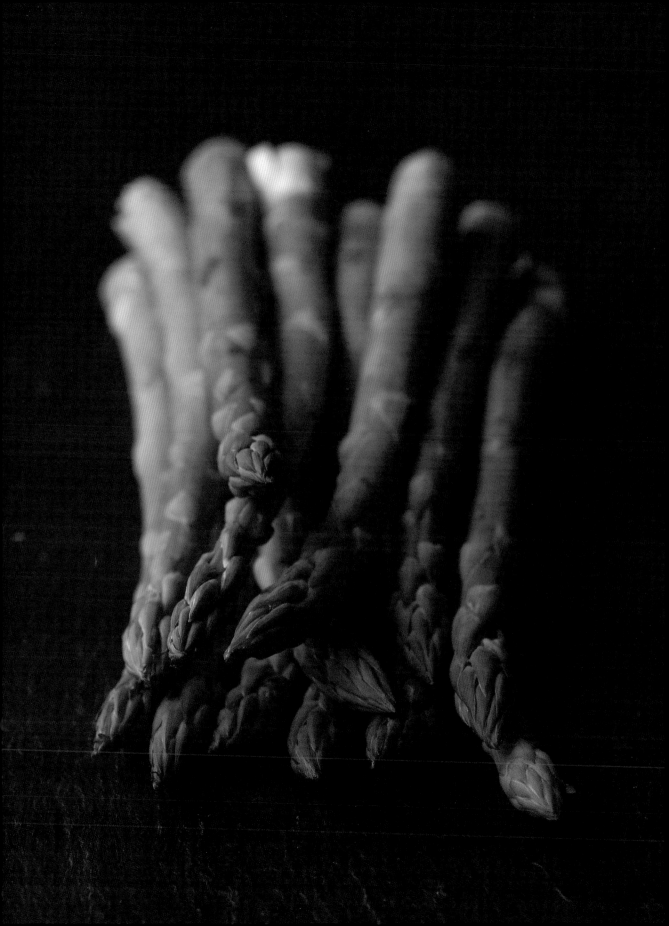

Avocados

Avocados contain potassium, folic acid, vitamin B6 and vitamin C, as well as lutein, an antioxidant that's beneficial for eye health, and vitamin E, which is great for healthy skin. You may have heard about the high fat content in avocados, but you should know that it is 70 per cent monounsaturated fat (like olive oil), which has beneficial effects on your blood cholesterol levels. (There's more about cholesterol on page 131.) Avocados have way more protein than any other fruit. The smooth buttery flavour is unrivalled and it's a great addition to your lunch box.

Selection: Haas avocados, which are nearly black in colour, are the most popular variety. Avocados ripen quickly after picking so be sure to check for soft spots. They ripen from the bottom up. Other varieties that have a firmer texture, making them easier to chop, include Pinkerton, Reed and Fuerte.

Preparation: Halve the avocado and remove the stone by poking a knife into the pit and twisting the avocado half. Peel and chop. If you intend to put it in your lunch box, squeeze a bit of lime juice on the pieces to avoid browning.

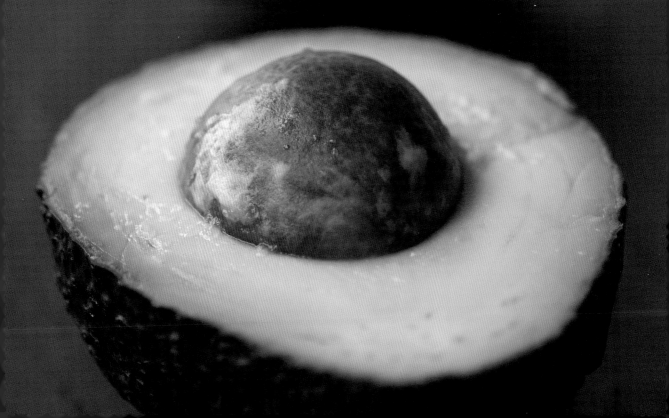

Broccoli

Broccoli is full of cancer-fighting antioxidants, B vitamins, calcium and iron. It's a fabulous addition to any lunch box combo and should be a staple in your fridge as it keeps well.

Selection: I tend to go for the broccoli crowns and leave the stalkier stuff for someone else. Make sure it's a nice deep green and avoid the yellowing (ageing) or pale green (lacking in phytochemicals) floret heads. Freshly harvested broccoli has smaller, crisper stalks and nice tight florets.

Preparation: Rinse well and chop off the large stalk. Cut the florets into manageable sizes and eat them raw in your lunch box. Steamed broccoli drizzled with a bit of olive oil is delicious with dinner.

Brussels Sprouts

The poor Brussels sprout has been ridiculed for years, but it is in fact packed full of nutrients and need not be a stinky veg if cooked properly. It contains decent amounts of vitamin C, beta-carotene, folic acid, potassium and fibre and a lot of protein as well. Potassium plays some very important roles in the body, including aiding proper kidney function and maintaining a regular heartbeat.

Selection: Make sure the outer leaves are intact and do not have spots or holes and that the cute little cabbage is nice and tight. Wilted leaves and a squishy feel are signs of poor-quality Brussels sprouts.

Preparation: To avoid the stinky sulphurs from tainting this delicate, nutty-flavoured cabbage, steam instead of boiling. Leave the sprouts to sit in lukewarm water for around 10 minutes to get rid of any bugs then steam them for around 12 minutes, removing the lid every few minutes to release the sulphur fumes.

Celery

Though not as nutritious as most vegetables, chopped celery adds a wonderful crunchy texture to your lunch box. Celery is a good source of fibre and is great at cleansing the digestive system.

Selection: Celery should be a pale light green. If it's bright green, it tends to be bitter.

Preparation: Simply lop off the leaves, rinse off any dirt and chop.

Cucumber

Cucumbers are 95 per cent water and add a cooling, crispy touch to your lunch box, even though they don't supply as many nutrients as other vegetables.

Selection: Dark green, heavy for its size and with no soft spots is the cucumber to look for. Shrivelled ends are a bad sign and, unlike some things, the smaller the better. Small ones have a better flavour and fewer seeds.

Preparation: The peel has the most nutritional value, so don't strip it off – just wash and slice away. I suggest cutting into chunky circles rather than thin slices so they maintain their crunch longer.

Green Beans

Fresh green beans are a true treat from nature. These crispy flavourful guys are fantastic for your lunch box either raw or lightly steamed. Green beans contain a good supply of nutrients such as calcium, B complex vitamins, potassium and beta-carotene and they contain polyphenols, which are great antioxidants.

Selection: Look for beans that are nice and crisp and devoid of wrinkles and spots.

Preparation: Rinse, snap the ends off and toss in your box. If you like your green beans steamed, toss in a piece of bacon straight from the fridge to flavour them. You're not frying the bacon, so there isn't any grease to contend with … just throw out the bacon when you're finished.

Greens

Drop the iceberg lettuce, which is nearly all water, and go for the wide variety of dark leafy greens. These powerhouses have loads of fibre, beta-carotene, calcium, iron, folic acid and chlorophyll. Some, such as kale, watercress, collard greens and pak choi, are also rich in vitamin C. The flavours range from peppery to sweet to slightly bitter. Mild-flavoured greens include collards, chard, pak choi or spinach. Stronger-flavoured greens include mustard, rocket, mizuna or turnip greens. Experiment until you find the perfect combination for your lunch box or buy one of the great pre-packed organic selections.

All dark leafy greens should be fresh looking. Wilted or slimy leaves are a sure sign of spoilage. Most greens are great just fresh, rinsed and raw in your lunch box. A few need to be steamed, as noted below. I've described the milder ones first with the stronger tastes towards the bottom of this list.

Collards: The stalks are inedible, but the round, slightly grey leaves are delicious steamed or sautéed.

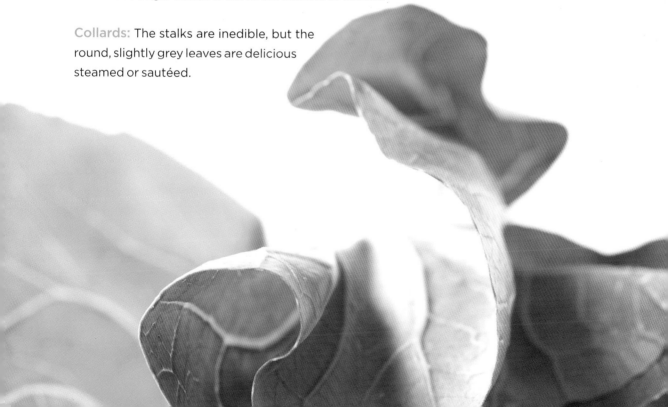

Swiss Chard: Chard is a gorgeous leafy green that can be red, green and even rainbow shades (pink, yellow and orange stems). It's a delicious as well as aesthetically pleasing addition to your lunch box. It can be eaten raw or sautéed and added to cooked meals.

Pak choi: Pak choi has a nice sweet flavour that goes well with almost anything in the lunch box but is especially good with stronger, more peppery varieties of dark green leaves. It can be steamed and added to a variety of recipes for dinner.

Baby spinach: Kids who grimace at the sight of spinach on their plates are obviously being tortured with that awful tinned slimy stuff that once gave Popeye the strength to overcome Bluto. If only Popeye knew how much better fresh, raw baby spinach is than that tinned stuff! Spinach should definitely be a staple in your fridge and in your lunch box. It blends well with everything and is delicious raw or lightly steamed.

Lettuce: There are many varieties of lettuce ranging from crispy romaine to oakleaf. Frisee's pretty white stems and curly leaves add a nice mild flavour to your lunch box. Mix with other more nutrient-dense greens for the best nutritional punch!

Radicchio: Red radicchio adds beauty and a nice flavour to your lunch box.

Tat soi: These funny spoon-shaped leaves have a good peppery flavour.

Watercress: Nutrient-packed watercress is fantastic mixed in with your lunch box. For a special treat, try watercress wilted in hot vinegar and olive oil.

Kale: Blue-green curly kale has an aesthetic appeal as well as a nice peppery flavour. Pick the stem and ribs clean, discard and enjoy the leaves. Try steamed or sautéed kale for dinner.

> 'Kids who grimace at the sight of spinach on their plates are obviously being tortured with that awful tinned slimy stuff that once gave Popeye the strength to overcome Bluto'

Dandelion Greens: Dandelion greens are a spicy addition to your lunch box. Slightly bitter, they should be added sparingly to enhance the box and not overwhelm it. Only eat the smaller leaves raw; the larger ones are better steamed.

Endive (or Chicory): Another frilly guy, endive is high in fibre and is another bitter green to add sparingly. Once cooked, endive takes on a slightly milder flavour.

Mustard Greens: Of all the leafy greens, mustard greens are by far the most peppery and add a nice sharpness to your lunch box. They become milder with cooking.

Rocket: The jagged leaves make rocket easily identifiable and the peppery flavour is wonderful.

Mizuna: Dainty mizuna with its lacy leaves graces your lunch box with a slightly exotic and spicy flavour.

Turnip greens: We'll talk about the root on page 67, but be sure to save the greens when you buy turnips. They have a sharp flavour that some might find a bit strong. Add sparingly, or try them steamed for a milder flavour.

Mangetout

Mangetout or snow peas are excellent in your box and another one of my favourites. I guess I have a lot of favourites! They are a good source of beta-carotene and potassium and because the pod is eaten, they are a great source of fibre.

Selection: These are awesome when they are in season. Look for vibrant ones that are crisp and devoid of marks.

Preparation: Rinse and toss in your box raw or steam lightly to serve with dinner.

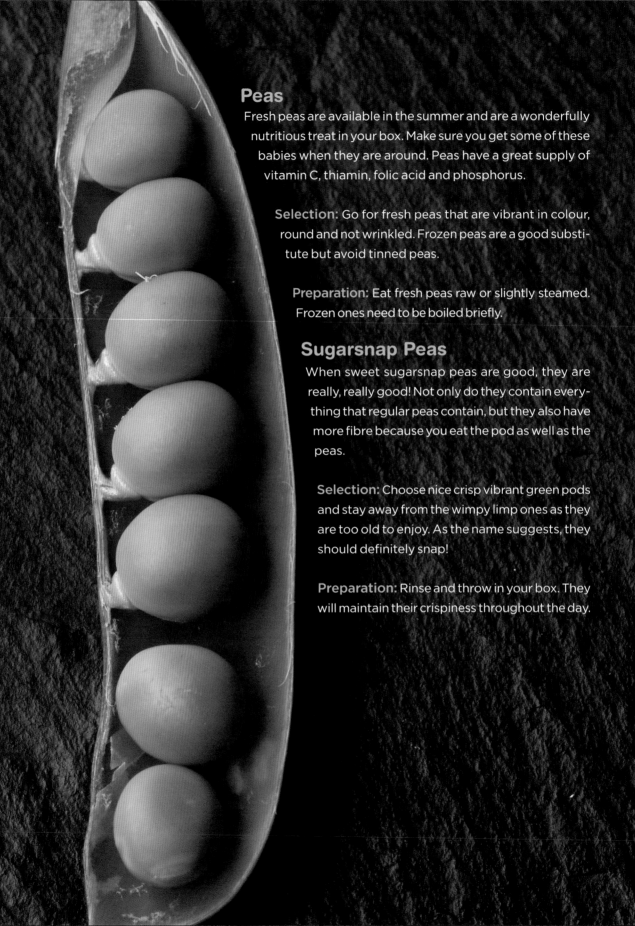

Peas

Fresh peas are available in the summer and are a wonderfully nutritious treat in your box. Make sure you get some of these babies when they are around. Peas have a great supply of vitamin C, thiamin, folic acid and phosphorus.

Selection: Go for fresh peas that are vibrant in colour, round and not wrinkled. Frozen peas are a good substitute but avoid tinned peas.

Preparation: Eat fresh peas raw or slightly steamed. Frozen ones need to be boiled briefly.

Sugarsnap Peas

When sweet sugarsnap peas are good, they are really, really good! Not only do they contain everything that regular peas contain, but they also have more fibre because you eat the pod as well as the peas.

Selection: Choose nice crisp vibrant green pods and stay away from the wimpy limp ones as they are too old to enjoy. As the name suggests, they should definitely snap!

Preparation: Rinse and throw in your box. They will maintain their crispiness throughout the day.

White

I couldn't think of any blue veggies but there are plenty of white ones.

Cauliflower

You can't go wrong with this mild-flavoured favourite. Its white florets last well in a lunch box and add a good, hearty crunch. It contains a decent amount of vitamin C and a bit of calcium as well as fibre and protein.

Selection: Choose a nice, tight cauliflower that has a good whiteness and no dark spots.

Preparation: Steamed cauliflower is delicious with almost any dinner and raw cauliflower is excellent in your lunch box. It goes well with most sauces.

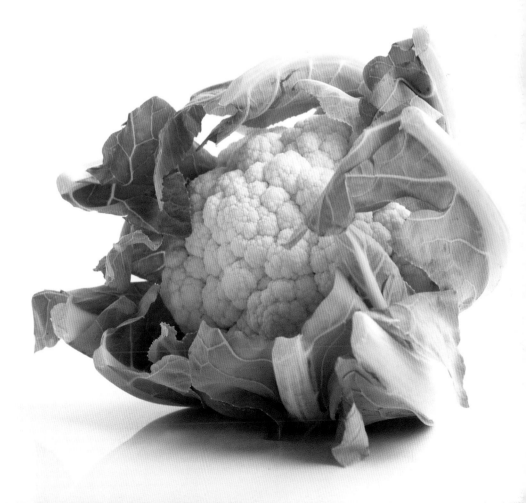

Leeks

Leeks add a mild, oniony flavour to any dish and have more vitamins than onions. Leeks contain lutein and zeaxanthin, which are carotenoids that play a major role in eye health.

Selection: Remove the outer leaves and clean well to get rid of any grit.

Preparation: Steam or microwave chopped leeks for about 5 minutes.

Mushrooms

Ahh ... the world of fungus! There are so many varieties of mushrooms available today that this part of the produce section looks like a woodsy piece of art. Mushrooms are good sources of three B-complex vitamins: riboflavin, niacin, and pantothenic acid. They are also very heart-healthy, containing potassium and selenium. Low in calories and high in fibre, you can't go wrong with fungi.

Mild-flavoured varieties include oyster, enoki and button. Shiitake, porcini and morels all have a more robust flavour while the beautifully coloured golden chanterelle is an interesting, fruity-flavoured mushroom.

Selection: Make sure the mushrooms aren't slimy and that their fragrance is earthy and never ammonia-like, which can indicate spoilage.

Preparation: Simply brush off the dirt with a damp cloth or rinse quickly. Don't let mushrooms soak as they'll absorb water. They can be eaten raw or lightly sautéed in a bit of olive oil, with onion, garlic and a dash of white wine. Mushrooms dripping with butter are delicious, but only on special occasions. I like to save mine for a reward alongside a fillet steak.

Parsnips

The parsnip is that vegetable that looks like an albino carrot and although it lacks its buddy's beta-carotene, it contains folic acid, vitamin C, iron and a decent amount of calcium.

Selection: The smaller and firmer the better.

Preparation: Parsnips can be used in the same way you would use potatoes. Sneak them into mashed potatoes for your kids or make them into oven chips as a healthier alternative to salty, greasy French fries. For your lunch box, cube and steam them.

Shallots and Onions

Keep a breath mint to hand for the sake of your work colleagues but don't omit onions and shallots from your lunch box because they have some pretty decent medicinal properties. They are strong antioxidants, and also have anti-microbial and anti-inflammatory qualities. They have been shown to lower cholesterol and improve renal (kidney) function.

Selection: There are many varieties of onion, so choose according to your taste. Red ones are nice and sweet, while white ones are strong, and yellow are somewhere in between. The skin should be tight.

Preparation: A neat trick for peeling and chopping an onion is to cut off both ends and make a slice down one side. Remove the outer skin. Cut a grid as far down as you wish to get the desired amount of onion then simply turn the onion sideways on your cutting board and slice as you would if you were cutting rings for a salad. Instant chopped onion without having to have the skill of a Japanese sushi chef! Shallots are a bit strong raw, but you can use them to flavour any red meat in your lunch box.

Simon's bite-sized tips

Onion Dressing

If you don't choose onion or shallot as one of your five vegetables, you can always chop or grate a little and add it as dressing.

Indigo/Violet

Aubergines

A good source of potassium and very low in calories, aubergines make a great addition to many recipes and are useful for healthy weight loss. The nutty, delicate flavour and meaty texture can be added to your lunch box quite easily. In Chinese medicine, aubergine is considered to be excellent for female health because it is believed to have properties that can relieve menstrual irregularities. Conversely, Chinese medicine dictates that pregnant women should not consume large quantities of aubergine due to the potential risk of miscarriage.

Selection: Choose an aubergine that is shiny and devoid of blemishes. Do not refrigerate but keep in a cool place out of direct sunlight.

Preparation: Aubergines can have a bitter taste, but if you sprinkle them with salt and let them stand in a colander for 30 minutes this will draw out the juices. Brush or spray them with a little olive oil and grill them under a high heat for several minutes, turning halfway through cooking.

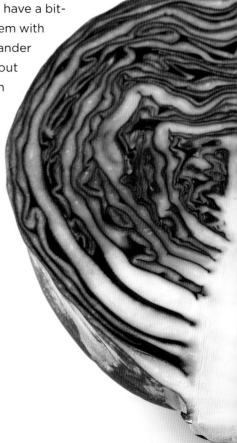

Cabbage

Both red and green varieties are nice crunchy components of a lunch box. They are good sources of phytochemicals, so long as they are not over-boiled.

Selection: Tight heads are the key and fresh-looking leaves are a must.

Preparation: Washed and shredded cabbage is ideal for your lunch box, but you should do the shredding yourself as nutrients are quickly depleted in pre-packaged varieties that have been sitting on the supermarket shelf. Steamed cabbage is a tasty accompaniment to the evening meal.

Turnips

Here's a great two-for-one deal. The gorgeous purple roots are delicious and healthy and the leafy greens are really great for you with vitamin B and C, potassium, phosphorus and calcium. Phosphorus has been known to aid in stabilizing metabolism.

Selection: Turnips vary quite a bit in terms of shape and size, but all should have nice fresh greens on top.

Preparation: Rinse and throw the greens in your lunch box. Peel large turnips and cook them as you would potatoes. Add them to your kids' mashed potato as a way of sneaking in a few more nutrients.

Using a rainbow of vegetables as part of your healthy weight loss efforts has many, many benefits. Pick one new vegetable to try every time you visit the supermarket or greengrocer. Before you know it, you'll be a veggie aficionado! Use this guide as a reference as you go down the healthy lunch box path.

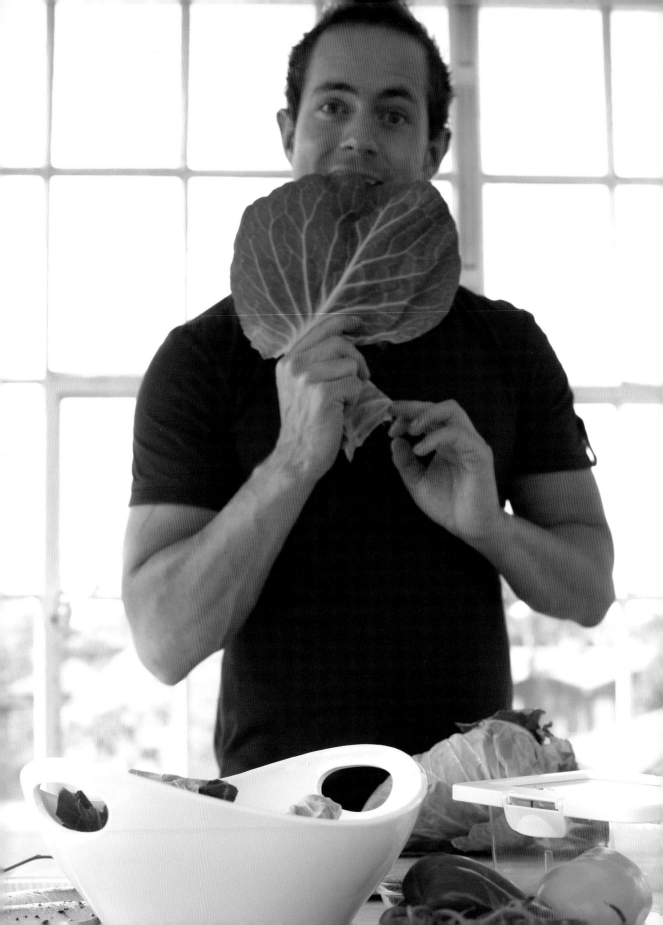

Why Fresh Is Best

As you've already learned, most of the food you will graze on in your lunch box is fresh. Almost all those vegetables should come from the fresh produce section of the supermarket rather than the tinned aisles. However, I'd rather you went for tinned vegetables than headed for the pastry counter. There's a reason for that. I want you to know what you're eating.

Potentially your tinned, boxed and bagged products also contain mono-sodium glutamate, butylated hydroxytoluene, xanthan gum or tartrazine. Do you know what they are? So do you really know what you are eating when you choose these items as opposed to fresh vegetables?

Listen, I don't claim to be some sort of expert on chemicals and the effects they have on the body, but I know they are not something I need to put in my body. Some scientists even argue that a small quantity of chemicals contained in any one food product can cause cancer or other abnormalities such as genetic defects. And if we choose tinned and boxed foods on a regular basis, that trace amount suddenly becomes a lot larger.

I realise why it's necessary to put preservatives in our food. Rotten food isn't appealing and it used to be the cause of a lot of deaths many years ago before we were able to preserve our food.

When your favourite vegetables aren't in season, you might have to choose frozen varieties or use tinned options. When you choose frozen veg, you should still go organic (see page 80) and low sodium (i.e. salt) if they are tinned. Some tinned veggies can be really high in sodium, which isn't all that great for your heart and circulation.

I don't know about you, but I was taught not to argue with my mum (I bet she's smiling when she reads this) and therefore, I don't think we ought to argue with Mother Nature either. The logic is that natural foods provide us with all we need and our bodies just work better with them. Unlike sugary cereal that has to have vitamins and minerals added to it to make it even remotely nutritious, fruits and vegetables are naturally healthy. So when you have a choice, why not choose fresh?

Group B: Protein

As you've learned, protein is a crucial component of your lunch box. Quite often, chicken breast is the first thing people think of when they hear the term 'lean protein source'. True, chicken breast is a fabulous choice for your lunch box, but there are also dozens of other choices that can be sliced, diced and chopped into your colourful container. Variety is the spice of life, right?

We talked about the importance of variety in terms of providing your body with optimum nutrition. The same holds true for protein sources and, in addition to that, it's important to keep changing your box so you don't get bored. So, let's delve into the world of protein and see what lies beyond the chicken.

Animal Protein

Protein is an important part of our daily food intake because it is the basic structural component of all the cells in our bodies. It's imperative for building muscle and healing the body, it's involved in the synthesis of hormones, antibodies and enzymes, it helps to transport nutrients and also assists in muscle contractions.

Protein is basically made up of chains of amino acids. Amino acids are the building blocks of all protein. The body can synthesise most of them, but some need to be taken in via the diet. These are known as 'essential amino acids' because the body can't make them and they need to be ingested through food.

Hopefully, I'm not boring you with all of this, but it's important that you understand why protein is so important in the diet. Without these nine essential amino acids, we'd have a lot of problems: we'd stop growing, wounds wouldn't heal, we'd experience muscle loss, lowered immunity and general weakness. You get some protein from the vegetables in your lunch box; however, the protein is incomplete, meaning that it does not contain all of the essential amino acids.

Animal protein is for all intents and purposes complete, meaning that it has all the essential amino acids. This is why being a vegan or vegetarian can be a bit tricky. Plant protein sources need to be combined with other plant protein sources to make sure that overall, the vegan or vegetarian gets all the essential amino acids. Once again, the trick is to eat a wide variety of foods, mixing tofu, legumes, nuts and seeds – so the Lunch Box Diet is pretty ideal.

Protein is fantastic but not just any protein source will do. Some protein sources contain an artery-clogging fat called saturated fat. I haven't talked a lot about fat, not because we don't need it but because you'll get the right fat in the appropriate amounts if you simply follow the diet. But if you'd really, really like to know more, here it is in a nutshell.

Saturated fats (found in red meat, cheese, chicken skin and so forth) are bad. So are trans fats (found in a lot of junk food). Good fats are unsaturated, and this is the type found in olive oil or avocados. The problems lie in the way the different fats are broken down in the body. Saturated fats get deposited in the arteries, promoting heart disease, whereas unsaturated fats protect against heart disease. Trans fats are the worst of all, linked to cancers and heart disease, and they are mainly found in manufactured products such as doughnuts, cakes and biscuits in which the original fat was hydrogenated (basically made solid).

If you want to learn more about all of this, make sure you check out chapter 8, 'Beyond Weight Loss'. For now, trust in the fact that I've already thought this out for you and though bacon's not on the menu, plenty of other good things are.

When measuring out a piece of animal protein for your lunch box, aim for a piece that's about 80 grams – roughly the size of a deck of cards. Start with this and adjust according to your activity level. If you are extremely active all day, you can have a bit more. If you have a sedentary job and your most strenuous exercise is going to the fridge to grab your lunch box, perhaps a bit less than your deck of cards size is in order.

Cooking and Preparation

Simon's bite-sized tips

Grilling is not just for summer BBQs. Whether on an outdoor gas grill or charcoal barbeque or an indoor appliance, grilling meat allows excess fat and oil to melt off and drip down through the grates of the grill.

When cooking eggs either poach or boil, or fry using a non-stick pan and a little spray of oil instead of butter or margarine.

Use monounsaturated fats such as olive oil or rapeseed. Avoid solid fats such as margarine, lard and butter.

Buy skinless chicken or turkey, or remove any skin before cooking.

When shopping for beef or lamb, choose the healthier, leaner cuts. Avoid marbled meats and go for the lean-looking bright red ones.

When grilling fish, it can have a tendency to stick so use a long two-pronged fork to carefully pry it off the grate rather than using a spatula or, worse still, tongs, which could break it into pieces.

Beef

Many cuts of red meat are quite lean. The best choices are:

- Fillet, sirloin or rump steak
- Topside or silverside roasts

Now, just because I didn't mention T-bone steak doesn't mean you can never enjoy one. You just shouldn't have one every day. You should also learn to eat less when you do indulge. Save it as a reward rather than as a part of your lunch box.

Beef is an excellent source of iron, which is necessary for the supply of oxygen to the cells and for a healthy immune system. Cut off any visible fat and grill steaks on a rack so fat can drip away. Roast joints without adding any excess fat.

Lamb

Though lamb is a bit fattier than other meats, it can be a nice treat to have in your box perhaps once a week after you really get going on the diet. There are many different cuts when it comes to lamb, and you certainly don't have to limit yourself to mint as flavouring (unless of course this is your favourite). Try spicing things up with black pepper or give the lamb an Eastern twist with cumin and turmeric. Roast lamb in the oven, using a rack to let the fat ooze out, or grill lamb chops.

Fish

Fish is a fantastic protein choice and you should aim to get at least two servings per week to reap the benefits. Oily fish, especially wild-caught salmon, trout, mackerel, sardines and herring, contain omega-3 fatty acids which can raise good cholesterol levels in the blood (see page 131 to find out more about this). Omega-3 fatty acids can also help arthritis sufferers and improve mood and concentration.

There are many different types, all of which have varying flavours and are suited to different cooking methods.

Simon's bite-sized tips

Raising the Salmon

Do yourself a favour and buy wild salmon rather than farm-raised. It's a bit pricier, but often contains much higher quantities of omega-3 fatty acids because it benefits from more algae. The free, non-farmed salmon is able to eat the smaller fish that have eaten the tiny fish that have eaten the little bitty guys that eat the algae – and the algae are where the omega-3 fatty acids come from. Farmed salmon may not always have the same diet. See? You can tell the difference between farm-raised and wild-caught salmon without even looking at the label: farm-raised ones are a sort of pale orangey-pink colour whereas the wild, line-caught ones are a nice bright red.

Tuna: Fresh tuna steaks are wonderful panfried in a tiny bit of oil or marinade, but if you're on a budget, tinned or the newer pouch versions of ready-cooked tuna are great. Choose fish that has been packed in spring water rather than brine. The flavours of some of the pouch versions can really spice up your lunch box but read the ingredients label to check they don't have added sugar or artificial nasties.

Sardines: Sardines are nutritious and can be a good time-saver if you buy them tinned in brine. They have a decent supply of calcium because you eat the tiny bones and they are a good source of omega-3.

Cod and Haddock: Don't ever be tempted to pop into the fish shop for the type that are fried in batter. Try baking them in aluminium foil with a bit of lemon juice and pepper. You'll soon realize that the fish alone is delicious without the grease.

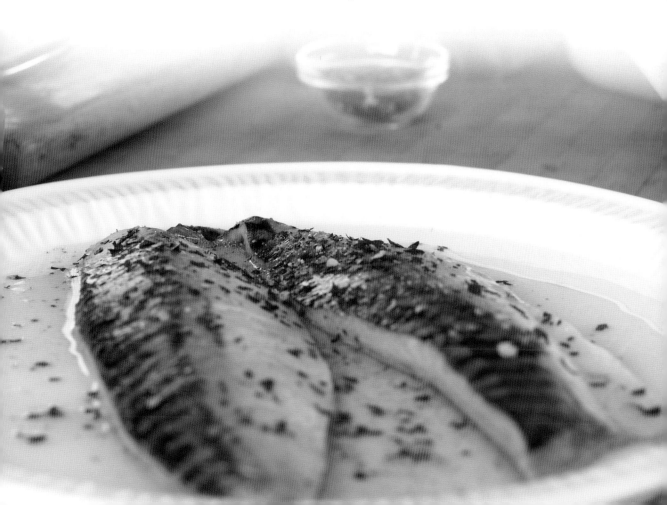

Mercury and Fish

Some big fish, such as king mackerel, shark, swordfish and tuna may contain methyl mercury. Mercury is suspected of causing birth defects and developmental delay in young children, so pregnant or nursing women and young children are advised to limit their consumption of oily fish. Other adults should also limit their consumption and favour fish and seafood that are low in mercury such as salmon, cod, haddock, mackerel, sardines, lobster and tinned tuna, as long as it's not albacore (white) tuna. Mercury builds up in the fish's system over time so it's the biggest fish that have the highest levels.

Swordfish and Sea Bass: Some of the best grilling fish because of their firm texture, these fish are also favourites because of their mild flavour, which is ideal for people who claim they 'don't like the taste of fish'. They are all versatile in terms of flavouring. One of my favourite ways is to marinade your fish for about 30 minutes in a lemon and olive oil-based marinade that has a bit of spice added in the form of chilli powder, cumin and paprika. After grilling, I dress it up with a bit of fresh salsa (see page 214 for recipe).

Mackerel and Trout: These stronger-flavoured fish are also good grilled. Mackerel's oily flavour is complemented by a tart taste like lime or lemon juice, and some serve it with gooseberries. The flavour of trout is slightly more delicate and can stand alone. Buy whole fish, cook them and debone them before tossing them in your lunch box – or buy smoked, ready-cooked fillets and flake them over your veggies.

Shellfish

Delicious and versatile, shellfish are an excellent choice of protein and heart-healthy omega-3 fatty acids as well as a source of zinc, iodine and selenium.

Prawns and Shrimp: When cooked without additional fat and served without huge dollops of mayonnaise, prawns and shrimp are good sources of vitamin B12 and have significant amounts of selenium and iodine. Frozen prawns are a handy freezer staple. They can be flavoured with citrus, garlic or, for a twist, try a shop-bought pepper sauce (but check the ingredients first).

Crab and Lobster: Crab and lobster are almost synonymous with large amounts of melted butter – but it doesn't have to be this way. Crab and lobster without the butter are incredibly low in calories yet high in protein and other important nutrients. They are also quite delicious with lemon and they add a nice sweet touch to any lunch box. Use tinned crab for convenience.

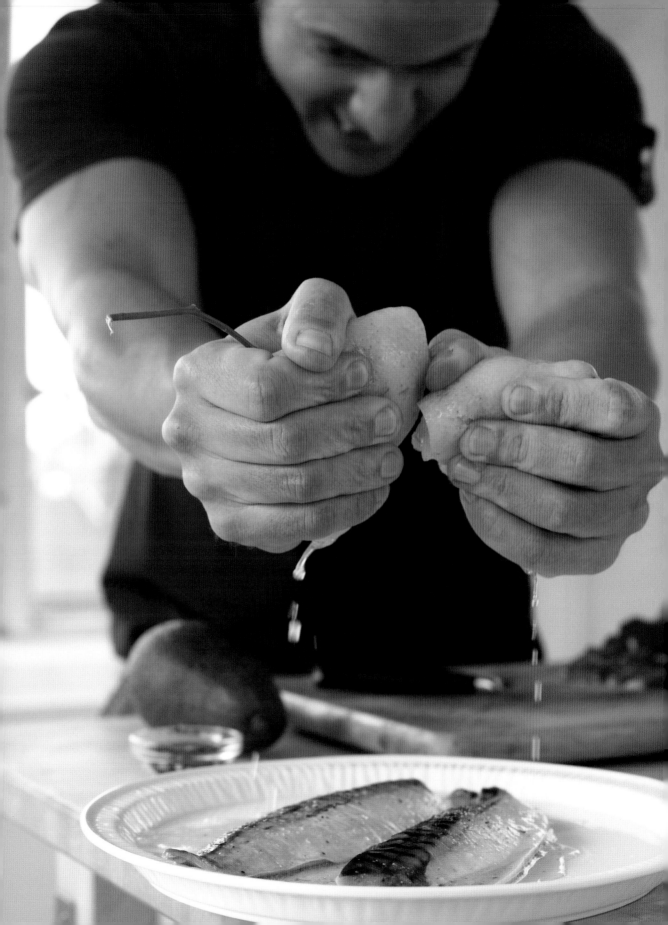

Mussels and Cockles: Mussels and cockles can be a nice change for your lunch box. Their chewy texture adds something a bit different. Scrub them, remove the beards and simmer them in a pan with stock and herbs and flavours such as ginger and lemongrass, or make a classic marinara sauce with tomatoes, garlic and basil.

Pork

'The other white meat', as the advertising slogan goes. Lean cuts of pork include pork loin, tender loin and centre loin – but avoid belly pork and crackling. An 80-gram serving of lean pork leg contains about 26 grams of protein as well as B vitamins, selenium, zinc and iron. Trim visible fat and roast or grill your chosen cut, saving the leftovers for your lunch box the next day. Pork is wonderful in a zingy marinade or served with a fruit chutney (see page 214 for a Mango Chutney recipe).

Ham and Gammon: Extra-lean ham is a relatively low-fat source of protein, but the problem with ham, gammon and especially bacon is that they are high in salt. Ham is one of those foods that is tortured and abused in the deli section of the supermarket. Look for ham that is devoid of fillers and added sugar and salt. Wafer-thin slices can be shredded over your lunch box. Gammon joints simmered in a marinade then cubed are a good source of B vitamins, potassium and zinc.

Chicken

Just because I've given you alternatives to chicken as a protein choice doesn't mean I don't want you to eat it. Chicken is a great lean source of protein and is highly versatile. At 26 grams of protein per 80-gram serving, a grilled chicken breast is a fantastic way to add protein to your lunch box. Put a few extra on the grill when preparing dinner for the family then slice them up and throw them in your lunch box the next day. Remove the skin before cooking chicken, because that's the fatty bit.

Because chicken doesn't have a super-strong flavour, it tends to go well with a lot of different sauces. Teriyaki sauce (see page 213 for recipe) makes a terrific marinade for chicken and adds just the right amount of flavour to your lunch box.

Because chicken is so popular, there are a variety of pre-cooked products not only in the deli, but in the frozen and meat sections as well. Go ahead and keep some frozen, cooked, skinless chicken tenders in the freezer but make sure you are purchasing real chicken and not some filler shaped like it. When you have these on hand, you can quickly toss them in a pan in the morning and warm them through while you fix the rest of your lunch box.

Turkey

Turkey is another great lean protein source. If you like, you can buy a whole turkey, roast and freeze the extra in individual bags ready for your lunch box. The night before you can simply toss a bag in the fridge and by morning, you have a delicious protein ready and waiting. Not everybody wants the hassle of that big old turkey, though, so check out the turkey breasts sold at the market or buy good-quality sliced turkey meat. Just stay away from the pre-packed watered-down stuff.

Like chicken, turkey benefits from a tasty dressing: try a Moroccan harissa paste or pepper sauce.

Eggs

When it comes to protein, the egg is one of the highest-quality and least expensive sources. A medium egg has about 76 calories and 6.5 grams of protein. Eggs also have vitamin B12 and a host of minerals, plus choline (a nutrient necessary for effective brain function) and lutein and zeaxanthin (good for the eyes). Just the thing if you have an exam or an important work challenge!

Keeping some hard-boiled eggs handy is just the trick for those busy mornings when you need to throw your box together in a hurry. You could even scramble up an egg to

Choosing chicken

If you don't already buy organic or free-range chicken, you might want to think about it. As well as having a higher level of omega-3, organic and free-range chickens are leaner than intensively reared chickens, as intensive growth and feeds have increased the amount of fat over the years.

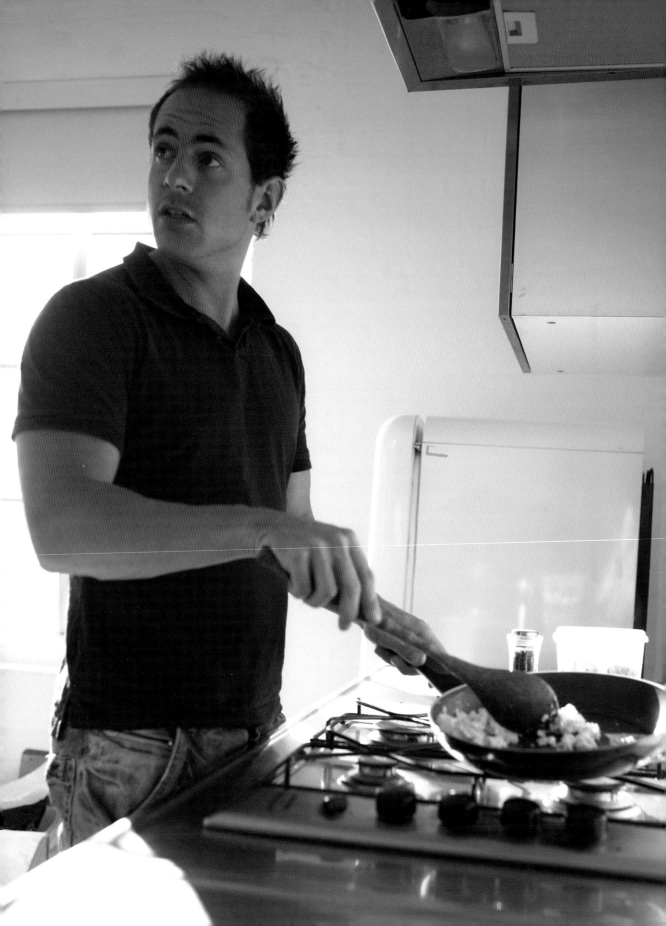

sprinkle in with your box (see page 204), using a non-stick pan or cooking spray instead of butter or oil. This may not sound very tasty but you'd be surprised when it's all mixed up with your vegetables and dressings! Poached eggs or omelette cooked with minimal fat are good choices for breakfast.

Plant Proteins

The Lunch Box Diet is ideal for vegetarians and vegans. I am a meat eater myself, but enjoy eating vegetarian or vegan meals for the taste as well as the health benefits. You might not be familiar with some of the plant protein sources listed below but do give them a try – you will be surprised how tasty they can be.

Because plant protein sources don't contain all the essential amino acids we discussed earlier (see page 70), it's important that vegans get a wide variety of these types of protein as well as incorporating wholegrains into their breakfast and dinner. You can also split up your plant protein choices, so that you have a bit of two different ones in each box. Just make sure to change things about so that you're eating different protein sources every day.

Tofu

Tofu is an easily digested protein that is basically curdled soy milk. On its own, it has a light, delicate flavour but it takes on flavour from foods it is prepared with making it easy to adapt to most recipes. Tofu is a great lean protein source that is low in saturated fat. Depending on how it is curdled, it can have a calcium content equal to milk. It also contains iron, phosphorus, potassium, B vitamins, choline and vitamin E.

I recommend buying tofu in block form in the refrigerated section of the supermarket. It can be cut into chunks, marinaded, then pan-seared, steamed or simmered with vegetables and seasoning.

Organic

Organic food has become quite the hip thing to eat these days. However, the 'trendiness' of organic food matters not. What matters is what eating organic can do for you and the planet. While it's not imperative that you choose organic foods on the Lunch Box Diet, I think you'll see in the end why it's best to choose them whenever possible.

We talked about not adding preservatives and artificial flavouring and colouring to our food. So, let me ask you this: if you can choose to eat foods that have never had pesticides, herbicides, growth hormones or chemical fertilisers sprayed or injected into them or that have not been genetically altered in a laboratory, why would you choose the other stuff?

Now, I realise that buying organic isn't always straightforward. Some areas have more organic foods available than others. I also understand that cost may be a factor, but there's a reason for that higher price which I'll explain in a bit. I also realise that there will be some folks out there reading this book who don't buy into the idea that any of this stuff is harmful to us or the environment. Personally, I beg to differ – and I'll tell you why.

To understand what makes organic farming so great, first you need to know a bit more about conventional farming. Conventional farmers can often use a myriad of chemicals and stimulants in the form of herbicides, pesticides, genetically engineered organisms and growth enhancers to yield their crops (and animals for that matter). By doing this, they produce large crops. Sounds great, right? Not so. In the process they also strip the soil of nutrients, not to mention putting all that muck on our food. Yes, some of it is washed off, but think about it this way. If I had two apples and you watched me spray one with a chemical and then wash it off while I simply washed the other, which one would you choose? Just because you don't see them spraying stuff on your food doesn't really make it any better, does it?

Conventional farming with all the chemicals and lack of planning for future soil fertility affects our health and our environment and the cost trickles down to you and me and eventually to our grandchildren.

Conversely, organic farming thinks in the long term by using proactive measures like maintenance and replenishment to keep the soil fertile. Instead of using toxic chemical pesticides, it takes measures like releasing predator bugs to eat the pests.

Translated for you and me, organic farmers produce safer plants, and in such a way as to preserve the bounty of the earth for the future. So thanks to them for all their hard work!

And don't forget the animals. As I've said, I'm a meat-eater. I know that this meat isn't graciously handed over by the animal before it skips away to live happily ever after. I realise that the animal is butchered for the sake of my food. People who are vegan or vegetarian have chosen not to be part of this process. I think that it's honourable and I commend you all for it, but I'm not giving up my steak. Many of us don't want to but what we can do is strive to buy meats that are organically produced.

Huge feed lots may hold a ton of cattle in less space than pasture, but what about all the disease that occurs? And in order to attempt to prevent disease, conventional farmers have to use antibiotics which may have an effect on the overall nutritional value of the meat. A lot of cattle are lost to illnesses that make their meat less valuable. Organic farmers don't use milk-stimulating drugs that leave the cows with huge distended udders. Sure, if you milk Elsie on the conventional farm more than Bessie on the organic farm, Elsie will produce more milk. But, in terms of overall health, ol' Elsie may give out sooner due to being overworked. Bessie will keep producing milk longer. See, short term versus long term. It's kind of like fad diets versus the Lunch Box Diet!

So chemically tortured plants and animals or pure foods from Mother Nature? Seems simple to me.

Pig Brother

Simon's bite-sized tips

When I was on Jamie Oliver's TV programme *Jamie Saves Our Bacon,* I was placed in a human version of a sow stall for over 20 hours. It was hell in there! Please please buy British pig meat where at all possible so you know that the animals have been treated well and are able to move around! Imagine if you had to live in a box for five years, as still happens in some pig farming outside the UK.

Legumes

Beans, beans and more beans. The legume family is a wonderful source of lean protein. Meaty beans can really add interest and texture to your lunch box. You'll not only be adding a flavourful protein source, but you're also giving your body a good shot of fibre as well as a phytochemical called diosgenin, which appears to inhibit cancer cells from multiplying. Beans are slowly digested and therefore stave off hunger longer.

I know I told you to steer clear of tinned foods, but part of the workability of the diet is quick preparation. Soaking dried beans may not be on the cards for some. Choose organic tinned legumes such as black-eyed peas, kidney beans, chickpeas (garbanzo beans), butter beans, aduki, flageolet, cannellini, haricot or pinto beans to name a few.

Lentils have many of the same health benefits as beans and add an interesting texture to a lunch box. Choose green or brown ones, which have more nutrients than red.

Seeds

Seeds are a great source of protein as well as minerals such as iron and calcium, which are both more difficult to get in a vegan diet. Seeds are also a great source of B complex vitamins, and vitamins A, E and D. Some good seeds with excellent flavour and texture are sunflower, pumpkin and sesame. Toast them in a dry frying pan to bring out the flavour. You can also try alfalfa, flax, hemp, poppy, linseeds and psyllium seeds. Some health-food shops sell interesting seed mixtures or packs of sprouting seeds. Sprinkle them over the top of your lunch box for a blast of vitamins and minerals. They can be considered the protein source or you can use them as the dressing if you prefer.

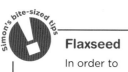

Flaxseed
In order to absorb the nutrients in flaxseed it needs to be cracked or soaked before use. Otherwise the seed travels through the gut and is expelled untouched.

Nuts

A little goes a long way in these nutritionally dense babies! Vitamin E, calcium, phosphorus, magnesium and potassium are some of the star nutrients contained in nuts. They are also a good source of heart-healthy monounsaturated fats. Just remember that because of the fat content, nuts are pretty heavy in calories and a serving is a handful, not a whole packet!

Some of the higher-calorie nuts are macadamia, pecan, Brazil nuts, walnuts and hazelnuts. Moving on down the chart, you'll find almonds, pistachios, peanuts, pine nuts and cashews, which are all very flavourful as well but a bit lower in calories. Choose unsalted varieties, of course, without any added oils or flavourings.

Coconut is high in saturated fat and comparatively low in nutrients, so apart from the trouble they are to open, I wouldn't go grating one over my lunch box. Chestnuts are extremely low in fat.

Vegetarians and vegans also get protein from grains, including the mighty Quinoa – a complete protein, which is very rare in the plant world. These are covered in chapter 5. But ultimately, if you are vegan or vegetarian the key to getting all of your essential amino acids is to eat a wide variety of plant protein sources.

That about covers protein. Whew! Better go take a few bites of my lunch box before moving on. You ... keep reading! You're about to enter the part of the box that gives all those veggies some spice ... sort of the 'G spot' of the Lunch Box Diet if you will. Now, now!

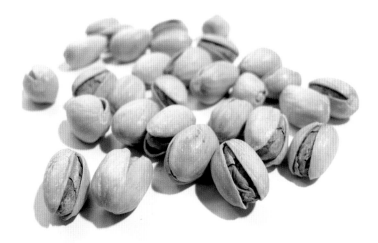

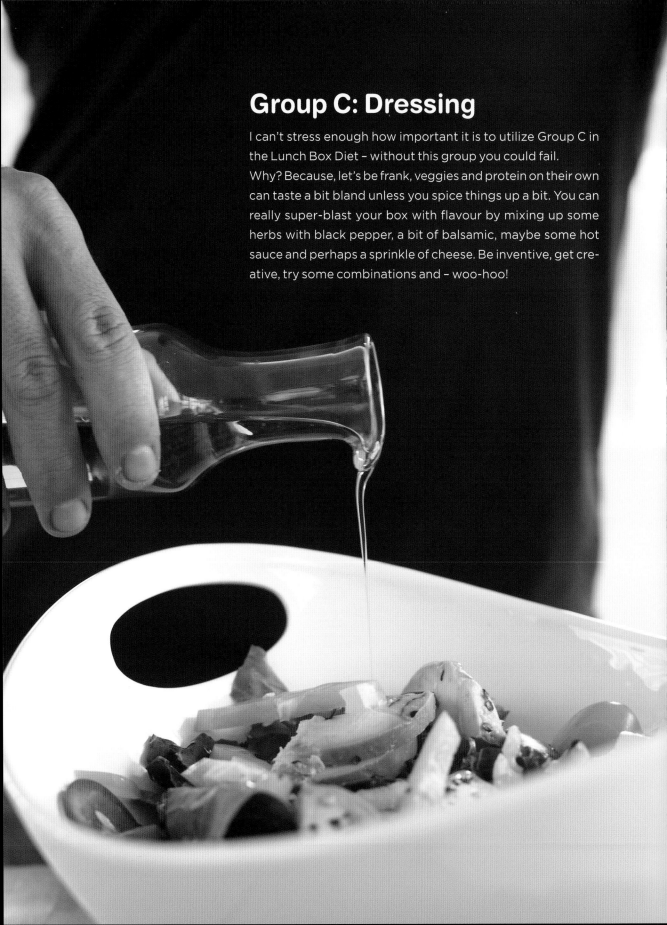

Group C: Dressing

I can't stress enough how important it is to utilize Group C in the Lunch Box Diet – without this group you could fail. Why? Because, let's be frank, veggies and protein on their own can taste a bit bland unless you spice things up a bit. You can really super-blast your box with flavour by mixing up some herbs with black pepper, a bit of balsamic, maybe some hot sauce and perhaps a sprinkle of cheese. Be inventive, get creative, try some combinations and – woo-hoo!

Oils and Vinegar

You actually only need a couple of teaspoons of oil to moisten your lunch box. Measure it out rather than tipping up the bottle and glugging, because at 45 calories a teaspoon, you don't want to go mad. The best oils are the monounsaturated ones such as olive or rapeseed oil, or delicious nut oils such as walnut. Experiment to see which flavours you like best. When using oil as the base of a marinade or sauce, remember the golden rule: **measure it out with a teaspoon!**

Vinegar is a fantastic way to add a lot of flavour to your box without adding a lot of calories. Balsamic vinegar is my favourite jumping-off point. Its flavour is fantastic all by itself and it complements fish, especially tuna, quite nicely. It is also great for red meat, pork and even chicken.

Don't forget about wine and cider vinegars, though, or fruit-flavoured ones like raspberry, which can add a great flavour to your box. The only one to avoid is malt vinegar, the type you get in chip shops, which would be a bit overpowering added to raw vegetables and salad ingredients.

Tomato-based Sauces

If you like it spicy, I've got a great salsa recipe for you on page 214. Avoid the jarred stuff you buy off the shelf at the supermarket which tends to have a lot of sugar and other muck added to it. Why? Probably to keep it on the shelf longer and also to cover up poor-quality tomatoes. Once you eat my fantastic fresh salsa, you'll never go back to the jarred stuff.

If you like a gentler tomato sauce without the chillies, spray a pan with a little olive oil, add a bunch of peeled, chopped, good-quality tomatoes, some garlic and herbs of choice (basil is the classic), season and simmer for 20 minutes or so until all the flavours blend in together. Make this in bulk and keep a jar in the fridge so you can add a dollop on top of your lunch box whenever you feel like it.

Simon's bite-sized tips

Basic Vinaigrette

This works with flavoured vinegars, wine or cider vinegars or balsamic, and with all kinds of herbs. Mix three teaspoons of oil with one of vinegar, and add a little mustard to taste, or a sprinkling of fresh herbs and freshly ground black pepper.

Raspberry Vinaigrette

Mix three teaspoons of olive oil with one of raspberry vinegar and add a little grated garlic to taste.

Loving it HOT!

I love spicy food and making my box hot is a must at least a few days a week. Ever wonder which peppers will add a nice sweet flavour and which peppers will burn a hole in your gut? Here's a quick guide to the varying degrees of this wonderful additive to your lunch box!

Mild
Sweet banana, Anaheim, Cherry

Medium
Serrano, large and thick Cayenne peppers, Chipotle

Hot
Long and skinny Cayenne, Piquin

Excruciating
Habanero, Jamaican Hot

Whoo, Whoo!
Bhut Jolokia ... (plan to leave work early!)

Hot Sauces

Connoisseurs of hot chilli peppers will tell you that it's an experience rather than a meal when you add the heat of really good peppers or pepper sauces to your food. So, unless hot peppers cause you too much trouble in the digestive area, I highly recommend you experiment with putting a little heat in your box.

You can use raw chillies to crunch on or a shop-bought pepper sauce (but watch out for additives). Tabasco, the old favourite, now comes in all sorts of strengths and with added flavours as well. There are also some great Jamaican jerk sauces on the market. The trick is to know which flavours and how much heat you really want. Check out the descriptions of peppers in my bite-sized box to help you decide which ones to choose.

Most shop-bought pepper sauces tell you what types of peppers were used, so you can either gauge your choices that way or by trusting the mild, medium, hot, very hot, 'your mouth will be on fire', etc. label on the jar. And don't forget black pepper! Do yourself a favour and purchase a pepper mill.

There's a rumour that really hot peppers promote a sort of euphoric state. Hey, I'm all for a healthy and safe way to take a chill at work!

Chutneys

Chutneys are wonderful combinations of fresh ingredients. Veggies, fruit and herbs with optional spicy extras make up tasty chutneys that can be added to your lunch box for an interesting twist. Some are a bit of a fiddle to make, so save them for days when you have a bit more time. Most will last a few days or more in the fridge. There's a recipe for mango chutney on page 214, but you should get creative and try out some of your own favourite flavour combinations. Sometimes oil is called for but be sure to use sparingly and make sure you substitute a good-quality olive or sunflower oil rather than heavy vegetable oils. Avoid shop-bought chutneys that tend to have added sugar, molasses or caramel.

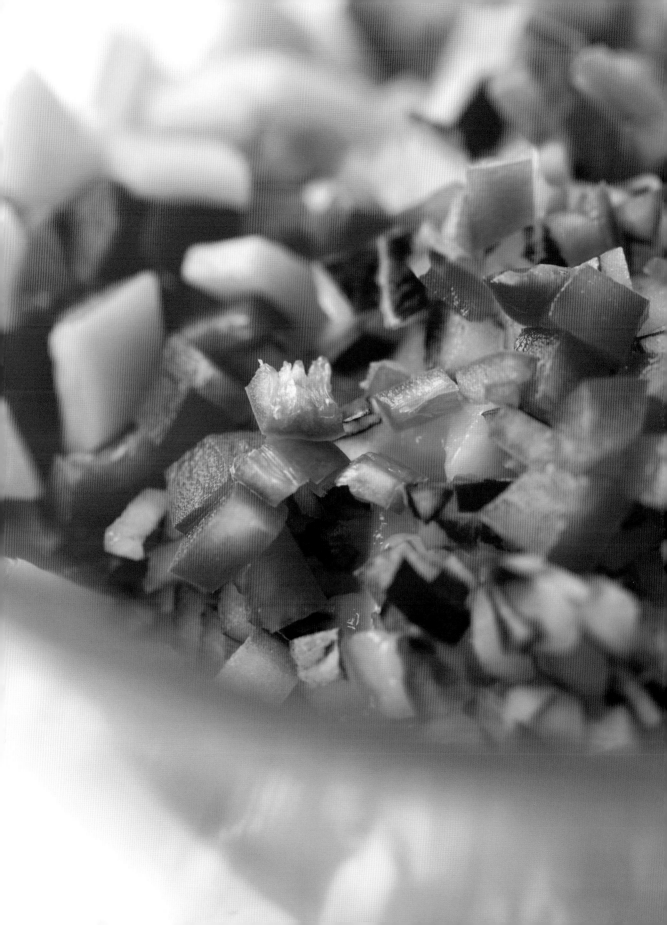

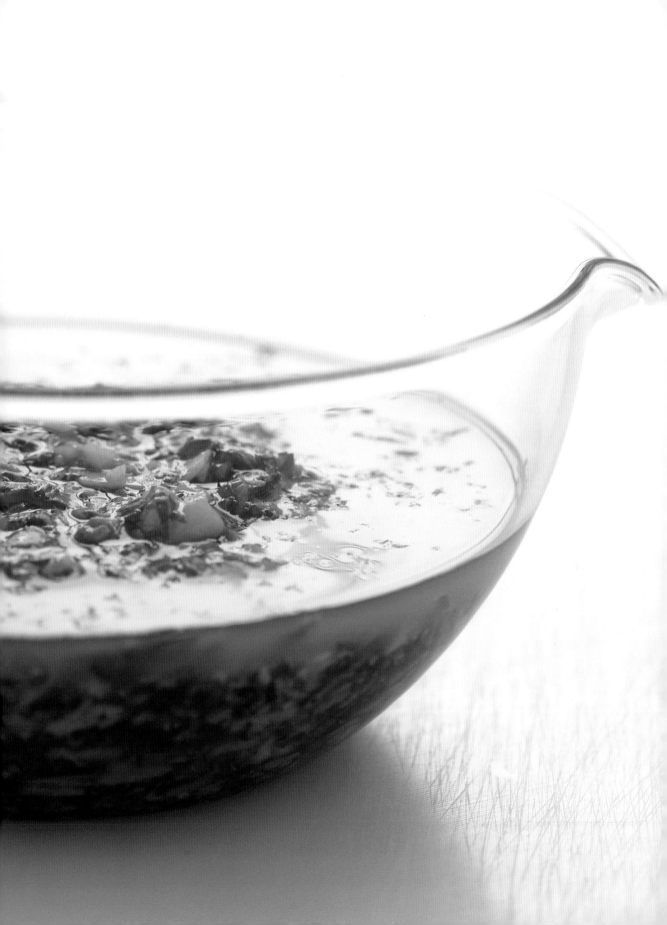

Fruits and Fruit Juices

One of the simplest ways to add flavour to your box is by squeezing the juice of fresh lemons or limes over the veggies and protein. Lemon tends to go best with fish, lime tends to be great on beef and they both go well with chicken depending on your preference. Orange and apple juice can also work with some combinations, if you want a little more sweetness.

While fruit should not be a major component of your lunch box, it can be used in small quantities for flavouring your food. It's sort of like nature's candy. Sprinkle some berries or pome-granate seeds in your box or a handful of apple chunks to add a little sweet flavour. Watermelon chunks are also lovely and highly nutritious.

In addition, some of those confusing 'is it a fruit or veg-etable?' items such as bell peppers and tomatoes can be used for flavouring. Roasted bell peppers and tomatoes have a lot of intense flavour that really spruce up the less flavourful veg-gies in your box (see the Red Pepper Sauce recipe on page 215). Sun-dried or sunblush tomatoes in oil are wonderful, as are olives. There's more about fruit on page 98.

Herbs and Garlic

Fresh herbs are great sprinkled over your lunch box. For a sweet additive, try basil. For a spicier variety try chervil, chives or summer savoury. Tarragon has an unusual anise flavour to it and is great with tomatoes – or try it sprinkled over your poached eggs in the morning. Coriander is great in oriental combinations, perhaps with soy sauce. Fresh herbs can be a bit pricy if you buy them in those little supermarket packs. They are, however, easy to grow indoors on a nice sunny windowsill.

Roasting garlic transforms its rather pungent taste into a much milder flavour. Drop a few bits of roasted garlic in your lunch box, give it a good stir and you'll find that a very little goes a long way. Don't forget the breath mints, though, for the sake of your colleagues.

Cheese

A tablespoon of low-fat cheese can be sprinkled over your lunch box, but avoid adding any oil when you use cheese. Instead, opt for pepper sauce or any of the other low- or no-calories sauces such as vinegars.

Any cheese is okay if you only use it sparingly, but low-fat varieties such as Mozzarella or Feta are best if you like the flavour. If you don't, use less of a higher-fat cheese that you enjoy or leave it off all together. What's important in the dressings section is to add tastes that you like.

My advice? Only add cheese here that will actually add flavour – and only use small quantities.

Marinades

Marinades not only flavour meat, but they can also be used to tenderise it. You can marinade chicken, fish and tofu as well. Most marinades call for some sort of oil, so choose olive oil and go easy. Measure with a teaspoon rather than glugging. There will be some kind of acidic component, such as vinegar or lemon juice, and then flavourings such as fresh herbs. Garlic is a good marinade ingredient, but go for natural rather than powdered, as it causes fewer digestive symptoms. Natural-yoghurt-based marinades are especially good for tenderising lamb.

Place your protein in a shallow dish and cover with the marinate – or, if you don't have enough to cover it, be prepared to turn every hour or so. Place in the fridge and marinate red meat for four to six hours, poultry for two to four hours, and fish or tofu for up to two hours. If marinating fish in lemon or lime juice or vinegar, be aware that this will partly 'cook' the fish. When they are finished, lift out of the marinate and cook as normal.

You'll find some of my marinade recipes on pages 212–13, but I encourage you to invent your own combinations based on your favourite ingredients.

Shop-bought Dressings

The ingredients to try to avoid in bottled dressings bought in supermarkets include:

- Sugar in any form (molasses, caramel, dextrose, maltose, glucose syrup, invert sugar and so forth).
- Trans fats (may be listed as hydrogenated or partially hydrogenated fat).
- High salt or sodium content (the new traffic light systems will show you when this is the case; avoid red ones for salt unless you will only eat a tiny little bit; high levels are 1.5g/100g salt or 0.6g/100g sodium and above).
- E numbers, preservatives and anything else that's not direct from Mother Nature.

Some good store-cupboard standbys can include:

- Harissa paste
- Horseradish sauce
- Soy, shoyu or tamari sauce (these usually contain caramel but not in high quantities)
- Thai fish sauce
- Tabasco or other types of pepper sauce
- Tapenade (olive paste with lemon juice and garlic)
- Mustard
- Vinegars
- Sauerkraut (pickled cabbage)

On pages 214–15, you'll find recipes for a number of sauces that could be shop-bought at a pinch, but the home-made versions are likely to be healthier. These include tomato salsa, tzatziki, pesto and teriyaki marinade.

You'll find more Group C suggestions when we get to the actual lunch box recipes in chapter 10. Bet you can't wait!

In some respects, my diet plan might be viewed as a low-carbohydrate diet. It is and it isn't, to put it as confusingly as possible!

Chapter 5

The Good, the Bad and the Ugly

The reason for limiting carbohydrate in the Lunch Box Diet is to do with working out what your daily calorie requirements are.

Again, no counting, but you do need to understand that if you wish to lose weight, the equation (what goes in must go out) must be adjusted accordingly without sacrificing important nutrients.

As I explained earlier, it's all about budgeting. If we view calories as money, then it can be said that we all wake up every morning with a budget of calories that will be spent on our food intake. Let's use 2,000 calories for convenience's sake, but remember that we all have different energy needs based on height, weight, age and sex as well as our activity levels. If you spend every penny of these 2,000 calories throughout the day but no more, you will maintain your weight. If you spend less and have some left over, you will lose weight. If you spend all of it and charge more on your 'I want a big arse' credit card, you will end up gaining weight.

So, when you lower your food intake to make sure there are leftover calories at the end of the day, something has to be cut from your diet. For optimum nutrition, will you cut out veggies and fruits? Nope. Will you cut out protein? Nope. Will you cut out junk that merely adds calories and no nutritional value? Sure you will! Unfortunately, this means refined carbohydrates, such as biscuits, crisps, some crackers, white breads, etc. – but with the Lunch Box Diet you should stop craving these foods anyway!

Remember that you can earn back calories by working out and generally being more active. When you increase your budget, you get to spend it differently. Much like life itself, if you make a lot of money per month, you're going to spend it differently than you would if you only made a little money per month. A little money only pays the essential bills just as a smaller calorie budget has to provide you with essential nutrients. A lot of money buys extras just as a lot of exercise racks up extra calories that can be spent on things that you enjoy more – but in moderation.

'Remember, you can earn back calories by working out and generally being more active'

Quite simply, a lot of the carbohydrates that most people consume are empty-calorie foods. Sure, they provide satisfaction in terms of flavour, and I don't want you to give up your favourites completely as you'll learn in an upcoming chapter, but in terms of nutrition, they do nothing for you. Imagine these calories as being like Monopoly money – it's not real, it won't actually help you to buy that house in Mayfair but it'll provide some short-term excitement. Then you're back to reality! Get the idea?

Remember, too, that all of those veggies you're eating all day are in fact carbohydrate, but they are the good types of carbohydrate. If you are a vegan or vegetarian and are using mostly plant sources of protein, those are carbohydrate as well. We'll be discussing breakfast and dinner in chapter 6, but they are mainly left up to you to create and will more than likely contain carbohydrate. If you are an active person in terms of exercise, whether that's because you choose to work out or because your job entails physical exertion, you are going to need some carbs to meet your energy needs.

Of course, this begs the question: which ones are the real and which ones are the Monopoly carbohydrates? You're just about to find out which carbs are the good, the bad or the ugly.

The Good Guys

Veggies, fruits and wholegrains are by far the best choices of carbohydrate and I encourage you to choose from these groups when you include carbs in your diet. They all contain fibre, which helps to prevent certain types of cancers as well as improving your blood cholesterol levels, heart health in general and decreasing your risk of getting type II diabetes.

There are two different types of fibre – soluble and insoluble – and both are important in the diet. Soluble fibre slows down the rate at which carbs are absorbed from the digestive system, making us feel fuller for longer. It dissolves in water and is absorbed into the blood stream, where it appears to lower

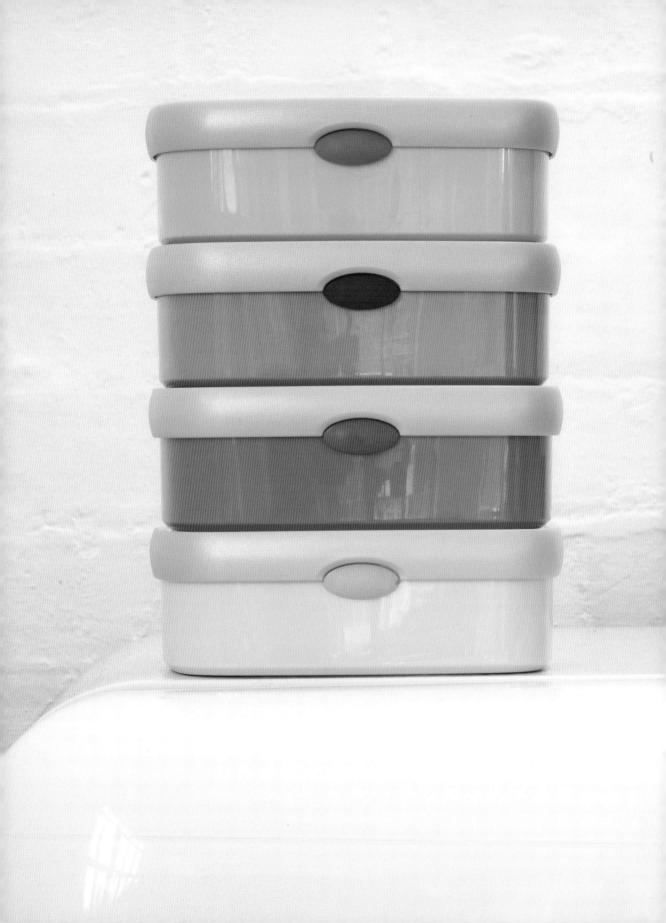

the levels of 'bad' cholesterol (see page 131). Insoluble fibre isn't absorbed through the walls of the digestive system but it helps to bulk things up and move food waste along, preventing constipation. When eaten together, they have an excellent cleansing effect on the body.

Your lunch box is a great source of both already, but when choosing carbohydrates for breakfast, dinner and/or as an addition to your daily lunch box if you are very active, choose either wholegrains or fruit.

Wholegrains

Wholegrains are really in the spotlight these days and because of this, many manufacturers are using the label 'wholegrain' or 'wholewheat' in their marketing campaigns. Be careful! There's a sure-fire way to find out if the label on the box means what you think it means. First, look at the ingredients. Wholegrain means that the entire grain kernel has been used, so in the list of ingredients you should see 'whole' oats, wheat or the like. If you see the name followed by 'flour', as in wheat 'flour', then it simply isn't wholegrain.

Another thing to check on the label is whether there is a significant amount of dietary fibre compared to calories. Shoot for 5 or more grams of fibre per serving with a total calorie content of less than 300.

Some simple ways to ensure that it is in fact wholegrain is to buy the product in a health-food shop. There you'll get bags or bins of all kinds of wholegrain products. Oatmeal is a good source provided it's the real deal and not a sugary, powdery type interspersed with a few whole oats; choose whole rolled oats instead.

Couscous (in its wholegrain form) is a fabulous, fabulous versatile side dish. You can flavour it with garlic and olive oil, hot peppers, red onion and bell peppers or any flavour combination you like. It's quick and easy and a favourite with kids.

Quinoa, a South American grain, is a useful source of all kinds of vitamins and minerals and has a lovely nutty taste. As noted before, it's a complete protein as well as being a grain and should be on any vegan's shopping list.

Good Carbs

Can be eaten regularly

Soluble Fibre Sources
Oatmeal
Oat bran
Nuts and seeds
Legumes
Peas
Beans
Lentils
Apples
Pears
Strawberries
Blueberries

Insoluble Fibre Sources
Wholegrains
Wholewheat bread
Barley
Couscous
Brown rice
Bulgur wheat
Quinoa
Millet
Wholegrain cereals
Wheat bran
Seeds
Carrots
Cucumbers
Courgettes
Celery
Tomatoes

Brown rice is also wonderful and you should definitely swap your nutritionally poor white rice for brown. Brown rice has a heartier flavour and texture that before long you will probably come to prefer.

If you like bread, aim for the nuttiest, seediest whole-grain product you can find. Aim for a fibre count of at least 2 grams per slice. Crackers and oatcakes can be high-fibre but read the list of ingredients and watch out for trans or hydrogenated fats (see page 131).

Fruits

A lot of people ask me why fruit isn't a bigger part of the Lunch Box Diet. It's not that fruit isn't good for you; it's just that with vegetables you get more nutrients per calorie. Let me explain. Fruit is sweet for a reason. It has a lot of sugar, nature's sugar, but sugar nonetheless, and that adds calories. Veggies don't have as much sugar and are, therefore, lower in calories. You can put a lot more vegetables in your lunch box than you could fruit and still have more nutritional value.

However, I always, always encourage you to choose fruit over other junky carbs like cakes and pastries! Fruit can be used in the Lunch Box Diet in a few different capacities. It can be a dessert after dinner or a snack while watching the telly. Adding some fruit to breakfast, whether it is complementing a bowl of wholegrain cereal or blended up in a smoothie, is a terrific idea. It can be used sparingly as flavouring for your lunch box. Sprinkling some berries over the top or adding a spoonful of mango chutney is perfectly acceptable. As a matter of fact, you'll notice that I even have some fruits listed in Group A of the lunch box categories, such as watermelon, avocado, tomatoes and peppers – yep, they're all fruits!

Bad Carbs

The worst category of carbs will follow, but these are the intermediate guys. The enriched and fortified versions of these foods have some nutritional value. They have been processed to make them last longer on supermarket shelves and also to be more palatable to the untrained tongue; however, certain nutrients have then been added back in. To understand what I'm talking about, pick up a box of kids' cereal and read the nutritional information. Parents see things like 'good source of calcium' on the label and allow their children to eat a bowl of sugar without realising it! Or, we pick up a box of crackers marked 'wheat' and think we are making a better choice than a bag of crisps. Well, you are and you aren't. Even crisps have a few vitamins in them but they only contain trace amounts of good stuff and a lot more bad stuff – some containing bad 'trans fats' (although to be fair many manufacturers have switched their fats) and sodium, to name but a few, as well as preservatives and additives which we'll talk about in the next chapter. And wheat crackers are roughly the same.

Am I telling you that you can't eat from this group of carbohydrates? Not necessarily. What I am suggesting is that on a regular basis, choose vegetables as the bulk of your carbohydrate intake because they are nutritionally dense. Choose good carbs for your breakfast, dinner and additional snacks if you are very active. Then, on occasion, you can choose carbohydrates from the 'bad' group – but I'm talking once a week rather than once a day. The next group is the one I'm most concerned about. The ugly!

Bad Carbs

Should be eaten rarely

Cereal made with
   refined white flour
   rather than wholegrain
Crackers made with
   refined white flour
   rather than wholegrain
Pasta and packaged
   pasta dinners
White rice or packaged
   rice dinners
Stuffing made from
   refined white flour
Non-wholegrain breads
Non-wholegrain noodles

Ugly Carbs

These are the carbohydrates that should be avoided most of all. That's not to say you can't indulge in a sweet or a bag of crisps now and again. We all have cravings from time to time but as you continue eating all the good stuff on the Lunch Box Diet, you will probably lose your taste for this category. Most of us have overindulged in the ugly carbohydrates for so long now that we have acquired a taste for them, which is why it's difficult to eat a bowl of fibre-based cereal instead of frosted flakes. It's also why we might not look upon a bowl of strawberries as a proper dessert, even though they are one of nature's sweetest treats.

The ugly group that I'm referring to are of course the truly empty calorie foods (remember the Monopoly money!). Aside from a smidgen of nutrients that have been added into the product, what you are eating in some biscuits, crisps, cakes, chips or lollies is saturated or trans fats mixed with sugar.

Worst of all is the nasty little trick that these empty-calorie foods play on your body. Unlike protein and complex carbohydrates, simple carbohydrates are digested very quickly in the body. When this happens, you feel hungry much sooner afterwards than you do when you eat proteins and complex carbohydrates. To boot, most of these foods are high in calories. One biscuit can contain anywhere from 60 to 150 calories. An apple might have 60 calories – but it will keep you satisfied much longer and provide nutritional benefits to the body. How often is one little biscuit enough? Don't you usually have two or three (or the whole packet)? How often do you eat an apple and go right back to the fruit bowl to eat another? Do you see the problem?

I get annoyed by diets that say you can eat what you like as long as you meet the calorie requirements for the day. Is that good for your body? Will bad choices give you energy and improve your skin, mood, and overall health? Of course not! It makes me mad that these plans aren't changing people's lives. They're a short-term fix because the weight won't stay off and

'How often is one little biscuit enough? Don't you usually have two or three (or the whole packet)? How often do you eat an apple and go right back to the fruit bowl to eat another? Do you see the problem?'

the vicious cycle will start again, this time with an unsustainable 'drink water and nibble a carrot' type plan.

I'm not saying you can't ever, ever have any of this stuff. You can. Now and again, just not every day. Sure, you could eat these refined simple carbohydrates full of junk in lieu of eating the good stuff and potentially still lose weight, depending how much of it you eat. But at the end of the day, how you feel inside is going to play a much bigger role in your overall health and enjoyment of life than what the scales read or the size label on your skinny-ass jeans says.

A lot of it boils down to retraining your taste buds to enjoy things that are good for you. If you continue on the Lunch Box Diet path, you will quickly find that your body realises how great it feels when you provide it with optimum nutrition and it will start to crave foods that are good for it. It will enjoy all the veggies and lean protein it gets during the day. When you splurge and eat something that isn't so great for you, your body will learn that there are consequences. Consequences like stomach upset, sluggishness and fatigue, or irritability that you take home to your partner. This all has an effect on the kids, of course. Are you beginning to see how eating properly can benefit more than just your waistline? It's time to get hold of what will eventually have a huge impact on every part of your life. Blimey – maybe you'll even get that new job with the higher salary. The sky's the limit once you begin to grow in confidence.

If you are a sugar junkie and it's too difficult to cut all of this out immediately, try eliminating foods one day at a time. Every other time you are about to pick up something sugary, replace it with a more wholesome alternative. If you're addicted to eating a bag of crisps in front of the telly every night, eat half a bag and replace the other half with a handful of unsalted nuts. Build up gradually and stick to it. Everything will fall into place and you'll thank me in the end!

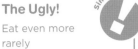

The Ugly!

Eat even more rarely

Biscuits
Crisps
Cakes
Sweets
Chocolate bars
Pastries
Fast food (such as pizzas, burgers, chips)
Deep fried food (fish and chips, fried chicken)
Full English breakfasts
Creamy, sugary desserts

If you are using the lunch box most days, you'll lose weight and feel better unless you are pigging out!

Chapter 6

What's for Dinner, Honey?

As you progress, you'll find that your body starts telling you what to eat. As it is learning how good it feels when it consumes all those veggies and lean protein sources, it won't thank you for eating junk for breakfast or dinner. I've put together some useful tips for those meals on either side of the lunch box.

Your Breakfast

Eggs

The good old egg has had a bad reputation over the years. But it is an excellent, affordable form of protein and I enjoy an egg-based breakfast almost every other day. Just make sure you don't take this great source of protein and mix it up with lots of fat.

Use a non-stick pan to cook your egg, or poach or boil it in water. If you like your yolks over-easy, you won't need butter or spread on your wholegrain toast (one slice) because you can simply moisten the toast with the egg. I like to sprinkle some herbs, black pepper and a pinch of grated cheese on top for an extra kick to the taste without increasing the calories like lumps of butter would. Add a small side dish of fresh melon or strawberries and you've got yourself a very satisfying, healthy breakfast that will tantalise your taste buds.

Cereal

If it has a toy in it, chances are you're not eating the right cereal! Read the labels and figure out which one offers the best nutrition per bite. Look for a fibre count of more than 5 grams per serving and avoid any added salt, sugar or flavourings. If you have been breakfasting on 'sugar crunchy o's' or something that changes the colour of the milk, you might want to make the transition more slowly with an in-between cereal, such as one of the grown-up cereals like Bran Flakes, Fruit 'n' Fibre or Weetabix . Then try some of the really fantastic cereals you can put in your bowl in the morning like rolled oats, muesli and wheat bran. Add some super-food berries, seeds and nuts to give you the kick you need – get your sweetness hit from fruit instead.

Smoothies

Smoothies are great for the morning rush. If you keep the right type of ingredients on hand, you're minutes away from tossing your breakfast in a bottle and heading out to work.

What should you put in them? If you junk it up too much, you may as well have had an ice-cream shake for breakfast – so follow my bite-sized tips. If you're buying smoothies, always choose ones with 100 per cent fruit content – there are some great brands out there. But it's best if you can make them yourself because you know exactly what's going in! Also, fruit starts to lose its vitamin content after it is juiced, so should be drunk as quickly as possible after preparation. Who knows how long that shop one has been sitting on the shelf?

Smoothie Ideas: Turn the page for some great smoothie ideas from one of my clients, Andy Elston, who has done fantastically well on the Lunch Box Diet and is always coming up with these fresh, energy-boosting fruit drinks. Try his ideas or invent your own combinations, using the flavours that tempt your taste buds, and see what works best. Be creative!

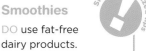

Smoothies

DO use fat-free dairy products.

DON'T use heavy creams or other whole-fat dairy products.

DO use silken tofu or soy milk in place of dairy but, once again, choose low-fat or fat-free brands.

DON'T use flavoured yoghurts that contain small quantities of fruit and large quantities of sugar and artificial colours and flavouring.

DO use plain (preferably organic) yoghurt with live active cultures.

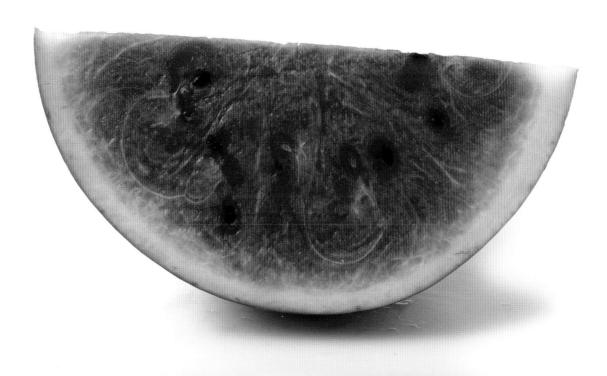

Smoothie ideas

Simply throw the ingredients in a blender and whizz for one minute.

Berry Booster

450g raspberries

100g blueberries

Juice of half a lemon

50ml fresh orange juice

Strawberry Blast

450g strawberries

2 bananas

50g mixed nuts

Juice of half a lime

Crushed ice

50ml orange or grapefruit juice

Hot Chilli Burst

450g raspberries

¼ bird's-eye chilli with seeds removed

Juice of 1 lemon

50ml orange juice

Your Dinner

You had a smoothie for breakfast and have been munching all day on your delicious lunch box. You walk in the door from a busy day at work and run to the fridge out of habit, but as you open the door you realise , 'Hey, I'm not famished!' Great! Now you have the time and energy to make a healthy meal. Even if you still have a load of laundry, kids' homework, baby's bath, not to mention your boss's presentation to finish, at least you have energy and won't waste time eating the contents of the refrigerator.

All silliness aside, dinner for many is a tough one. You've got a leg up on the situation by eating healthily all day, but what about the rest of the family? They may not think an 80g piece of salmon and a side salad are going to be enough. Then, there's always the partner who will look at your lovingly pre-pared spring green salad and ask you why you're serving weeds to the family.

No worries. I'm here to help. I'm going to give you some ideas that are not only healthy for you, but healthy and work-able for the rest of the family. Besides, it's time they join the club and get on board with your healthy endeavours!

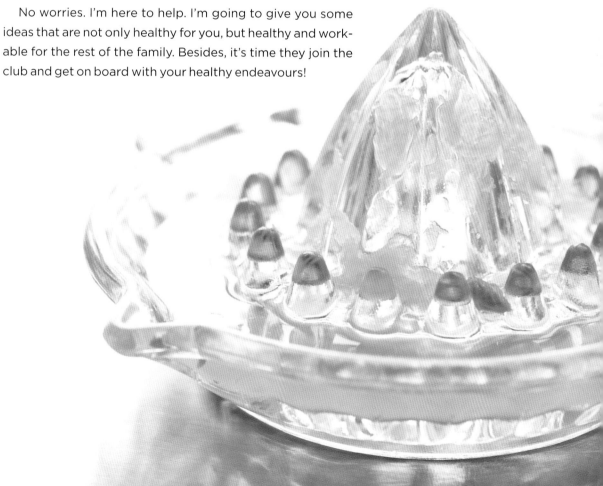

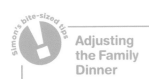

simon's bite-sized tips

Adjusting the Family Dinner

To swap starchy accompaniments for healthier ones:

Mix white rice with brown rice and change the proportions until it's eventually all brown rice.

Use parsnips in your mashed potatoes and prepare them with chicken stock instead of milk.

Swap white pasta for wholegrain pasta and add some fresh herbs for flavour instead of heavy cream sauces.

Choose wholegrain couscous as a wonderful alternative to packaged rice dinners. Flavour it with herbs and vegetables.

Try quinoa for a change. This nutty-flavoured grain is high in protein and an excellent source of fibre.

Millet is a fabulous wholegrain that can be added to soups and stews or used as a stuffing.

Opt for wholegrain instead of white rolls.

Reinventing the Family Meal

Traditionally, many of us view dinner as meat with rice or potatoes, possible one or two boiled veggies, a side plate of bread and butter, and a creamy or sugary dessert to finish. And if we do have any salad, it's covered wth creamy dressing.

We eat this way because it's how we were raised. It's traditional to have a big meal in the evening, but not necessary. The first day you begin the Lunch Box Diet, you will notice that you aren't nearly as hungry at dinner time. You have taken in most of your daily nutrient requirement already, so you don't need a big 'balanced' meal at the end of the day.

A lot of what we deem 'necessary' at dinner time is merely filler. All of those flavourful, starchy sides like mashed potatoes, pasta, noodles and stuffing can be enjoyable yet I think their real purpose is to make the meal stretch a bit. Though your stomach is being retrained via grazing all day, your family is still used to this traditional meal.

Remember that a serving of meat should be around 80 grams. That's about the size of a deck of cards. Not a lot, right? We're so used to putting a big old hunk of meat on our plates and filling the rest with starch that we don't realize how very little we need. Your family might need a bit more than you so don't expect them to give up their huge portions and starchy accompaniments all at once.

As you have already learned, fresh, raw and/or lightly steamed or microwaved vegetables are far better for you than tinned or boiled ones. If your family is used to soggy cauliflower soaked in cheese sauce, it may take them a bit of time to get used to eating the good stuff. Just as you are retraining your taste buds, they will learn over time to enjoy veggies in a more natural state.

Your Kids

In a world where levels of childhood obesity are increasing, I couldn't possibly leave the welfare of youngsters out of my book. I used to be an overweight kid and I know how hard it is.

First of all, know this: **it all begins with you.** When Dorothy Law Nolte wrote a poem entitled 'Children learn what they live', she couldn't have been more correct. You can spend days on end preaching to your child about what they should or should-n't do, but what they see you doing has a far greater impact. When you eat well and take good care of your body, your children will learn what they live. When they see Mum and Dad exercise they tend to copy this behaviour. When you practise good eating habits at the dinner table, you are helping your children to learn valuable lessons about good nutrition.

'First of all, know this: it all begins with you'

Portions and Grazing

You might think that your child needs a lot of food because they are growing, and so you load their plates. However, large meals and large portions are likely to cause unhealthy weight gain either now or down the line. Just like you, children can train their stomachs to expect more or less food.

Children are natural grazers, wandering into the kitchen say-ing 'Mummy, I'm starving!' only two hours after they've eaten lunch. However, if they get accustomed to three huge meals and then snacks in between, this is where the trouble will begin. Instead, gradually offer smaller portions at their main meals; they probably won't even notice. For the day, keep a wide array of healthy snacks on hand: ready-chopped vegetable crudités and fresh fruit sticks in the fridge; trail mix; celery sticks to dip into natural peanut butter; wholegrain cereals.

If children are at home all day, you could make them their own lunch box. Start by letting them help you to prepare your box and ask them if they'd like to try a bite. Allow them to pick what they want, but if they keep choosing the meat, ask them to try at least one veggie. Before long you may find that they are begging to have their own box.

No Dinner Date?

When you're on your own surely there's no excuse for not having a healthy dinner? Or is there? What about the On-the-Run Dinner: 'Yes, I want fries with that, super-size it and hurry up… I'm on my way to the club!' Or the Evening-at-Home Dinner: leftover pizza, crisps and a cream cake.

Switching to a more healthy dinner doesn't have to be difficult. When it comes to convenience food, it can be hard to find anything that isn't loaded with junk and devoid of nutritional value, but if you are creative enough, it can be done.

First, there's the deli – some use organic produce, free of artificial sweeteners, colouring, flavouring and synthetic preservatives. Less healthy delis offer tray after tray of fried foods and mystery meats. If you must, opt for chicken breast or salads that haven't any added dressing.

Another option is an open sandwich with a good-quality cold meat, a little cheese, salad and some seasonings such as vinegar or herbs. Use good-quality wholegrain bread as a base for your masterpiece but eliminate that extra piece of bread on top. Keep it open!

How about a cold plate? You can have a colourful platter of raw veggies, fruit, good-quality deli meat, wholegrain crackers and low-fat cottage cheese.

Now, what about restaurants? First of all, you'll have a lot of trouble eating healthily in a fast-food joint. Most of the salads are nothing more than iceberg lettuce accompanied by horrendously creamy dressing. Spinach salads with grilled chicken are a pretty decent choice, but make sure you skip the dressing and opt for a lemon wedge instead, or bring your salad home and use your own homemade vinaigrette.

If you're dining in a restaurant, don't be afraid to ask how dishes are prepared. Ask that they skip the added butter when grilling your fish and leave the cream sauce in the kitchen. Opt for roasted or steamed veggies instead of potatoes.

And, if you're out for your birthday then enjoy it! It's only once a year and you can get back on the right track the next day.

Simon's bite-sized tips

Pizza

Instead of ordering pizza try this. Buy a wholegrain pizza crust, spread it with a thin layer of olive oil then sprinkle on some spinach, rocket, radicchio, chopped red onion, peppers, fresh tomatoes and chunks of marinated grilled chicken breast. Then add a light sprinkling of low-fat mozzarella. Follow the directions on the pizza crust packaging for baking temperature and time.

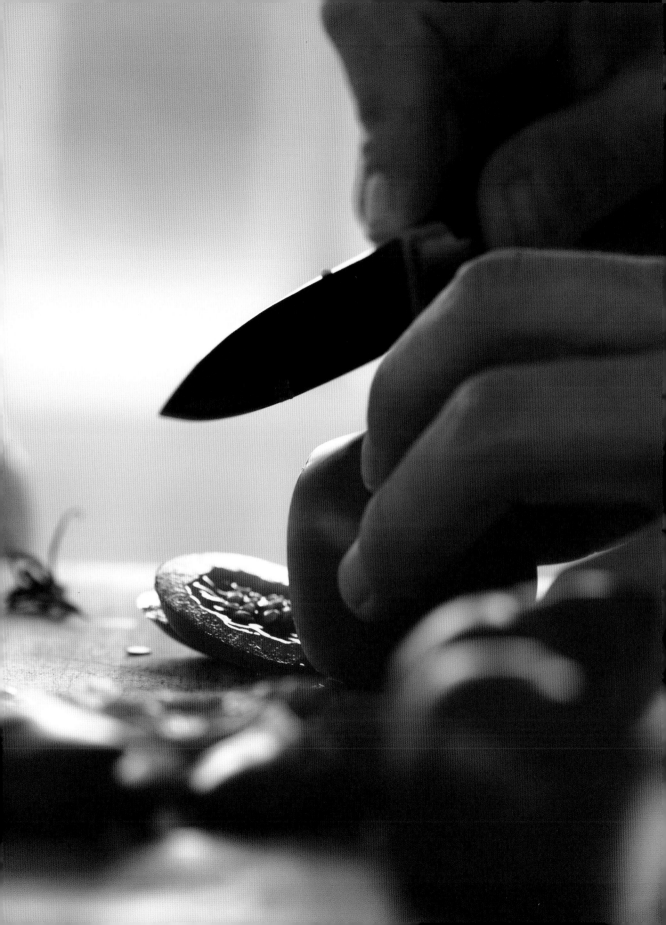

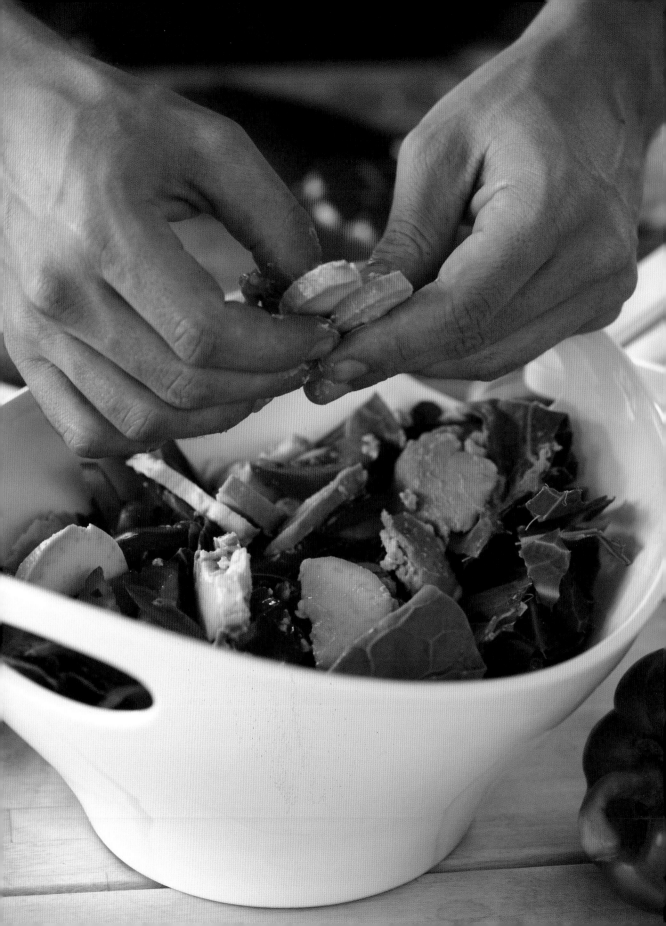

Cooking for Yourself

Make sure you have the right ingredients in your fridge and store cupboard. Keeping a well-stocked kitchen may not be high on your priority list but in the end it will save you loads of time and frustration. There's nothing more annoying than beginning a recipe and finding you're short of an ingredient. Plan ahead and have a menu in mind for the coming week or at least the next few days.

I have a little saying for my clients that I call the 5 Ps:

Poor Planning Promotes Poor Performance

Think ahead to your lunch box as well as evening meals and you'll be less likely to grab unhealthy snacks when you're hungry. Prepare some extra vegetables or protein for your lunch box the next day.

Plan ahead and take a shopping list to the supermarket. Over time, you'll build up a pretty good stock of foods and will be able to create many recipes at the last minute.

What should you cook? Here's an idea for a typical dinner – grilled wild salmon with roasted red peppers, spring salad, couscous flavoured with garlic and olive oil and, for dessert, a bowl of strawberries.

You can then try mixing things up a bit by swapping the ingredients with some of the other fantastic flavours and ingredients that we looked at earlier in chapter 4. For example, try using chicken or tuna instead of wild salmon, and other vegetables, such as aubergines or sweet potatoes, instead of red peppers, and a different fruit for dessert. Don't forget to make a little extra fish or meat that you can put in your lunch box the next day. There are so many variations – before you know it, you've got all your meals and lunch boxes planned for the whole week.

Simon's bite-sized tips

Beef Wrap

Before you leave in the morning, throw together the Spicy Beef Marinade (see page 212) and marinade some strips of top sirloin throughout the day. When you get home, grill the strips along with some peppers, tomatoes and onions. Mix them all up and roll them in a wholegrain tortilla. Make some extra so that you can throw it into a lunch box the next day.

Are You Going to Cheat on Me?

I'm not telling you that you can eat whatever you want. That would be preposterous and is the stuff of make-believe fad diets that never, ever work.

If you want a fairy tale, you're reading the wrong book. But if you want a satisfying meal plan that will still allow you to lose weight, read on!

If you've already begun the diet, you're probably realising that the temptation to eat junk is lessening on a daily basis. Once you get going you'll realise a very important aspect of optimum nutrition: it makes you feel so good that the feeling is better than any of those unhealthy tastes you once craved.

I know that you're not going to cheat on me too badly. Nevertheless, let's talk about indulgences. These aren't strictly off limits. Make a list of all the foods you consider to be your 'weaknesses'. I want you to be aware of these items and learn how and when to eat them.

I believe strongly that every time we deny ourselves something we truly enjoy, say chocolate, we drop a little pebble in the binge bucket. Am I saying you should give in to every urge? No. Sorry. As I mentioned earlier, we often use these comfort foods to camouflage and mask emotional pain. So if you find yourself reaching for these yummy little no-no's a lot, re-read chapter 2.

But we don't always have to have a deep emotional reason for eating a doughnut. Sometimes, a doughnut is just a doughnut. If you constantly deny yourself things you truly love, all those pebbles you're dropping into the binge bucket are going to start spilling over and you'll end up eating an entire carton of doughnuts or a box of chocolates.

If chocolate was one of the items on your list, rather than buying a whole box, buy a single hand-made truffle and enjoy it after your dinner tonight. If you are craving crisps, opt for the snack-size bag instead of the large family pack and enjoy! Eat slowly and enjoy your treat. You deserve it! You're eating healthily most of the time now, so having a little yummy now and again is absolutely okay.

'Optimum nutrition makes you feel so good that the feeling is better than any of those unhealthy tastes you once craved'

I spoke earlier about 'earning' food. The same principle applies here. If you're working out and following a healthy diet, then there's no reason why you can't have a sweet treat or a salty snack. Depending on how much you work out and how well you eat the rest of the day, you might even be able to have a treat every day. You see? Eating vegetables and lean protein most of the time leads to weight loss which is enhanced by working out, which allows you to have a few indulgences now and again.

How to Avoid Cheating

- When you're feeling really down, don't automatically reach for food. Go for a walk, call a friend, read a book or watch a movie.
- If you're the type to eat while watching the telly, do some sort of mindless task like ironing or sewing while your favourite show is on. This will keep your hands busy.
- Tip out a small portion of your snack into a bowl rather than taking the entire bag to the sofa with you. You're far less likely to get carried away.
- Try not to overload your fridge and cupboards with junk. Avoid buying tons of yummy treats for the kids. They don't need a lot of that stuff either and it's going to be tempting for you. Stave off temptation by not keeping much (if any) 'treat food' in the house in the first place.

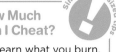

How Much Can I Cheat?

You earn what you burn, so how much can you cheat?

- 'I get up to change the television channel instead of using the remote.'

Don't cheat more than once a week.

- 'I work out two or three times a week but have a sedentary job.'

You can cheat a couple of times a week.

- 'I'm a busy mum who chases children all day and works out two or three times a week.'

Cheat a little three to four times a week.

- 'I love to work out. I'm at the gym two hours every day sweating profusely!'

If you work out for even 40 minutes most days of the week, you can probably indulge in a treat every evening and get away with it.

About 55 to 60 per cent of the human body is water. Proper cellular function relies on adequately hydrated tissue so keeping your body hydrated is essential for optimum health

Chapter 7
Thirsty?

There are loads of sports drinks, flavoured waters, teas and juices out there, but how much and what should you be drinking? Fluid requirements are around 1 ml of water per calorie consumed. This is on average around 2 litres per day. Picture a 2-litre container of water: this is roughly how much you should aim to drink throughout the day, though not all at once. There are certain factors that increase this need, such as sun exposure and working out. All that sweating depletes your body of fluid, and dehydration can set in more quickly. You will also have higher fluid requirements if you live in a dry climate and/or a higher altitude. Fluid requirements also increase with illness so remember to drink up when you have flu or colds, especially if you have a fever.

Once you become thirsty, you are already partially dehydrated. Avoid this by getting into the habit of sipping throughout the day.

You don't have to get all your fluid requirements from water alone. The fluid content in other beverages you consume counts as well, as does the fluid content of your vegetables. Water is very good for you, though, so I would suggest that you aim to drink a litre of it a day, and top up the rest with some other alternatives, as described in the rest of this chapter.

Water

We'll start with water because it is by far the best source of fluid for your body. I've often said that I wish I was the bloke who'd thought of bottling water. Something we once thought of as 'free' can now cost a pretty penny per bottle.

With all of the gunk that's added to our water supply, I'm not convinced that bottled water is merely a convenience. A lot of people swear they can't bear to drink tap water any more because of the impure taste compared to bottled water. Whether or not your bottled water advertises that it came from the 'pure springs of the hills of whatever', chances are it is much cleaner than your city tap water. But you don't need to spend a ton of money to make sure the water you're consuming is safe.

First, consider spending the money up front. You can get reverse osmosis systems installed under your kitchen sink to filter out all the impurities in your water, or buy a filter jug. Some refrigerators are equipped with water and ice dispensers and these usually have some sort of filtering system. Ultimately, it's worth buying some kind of filtration system as it will work out cheaper than continually forking out for bottles of mineral water.

Flavoured Waters

Mineral waters, vitamin waters, waters that promise to make you clever ... it seems this section of the market is growing and growing. Some of these pumped-up waters aren't bad choices but make sure you read the label and see for yourself if it has a ton of calories from added sweeteners, and consider whether it really has the vitamins and minerals it claims in order to justify the calories.

Remember, if you're following the Lunch Box Diet, you are already getting your full daily requirement of vitamins and minerals so this hyped-up water isn't necessary. However, if you like it, it's definitely better than a cola or other sugary drinks.

> **Simon's bite-sized tips**
>
> **Water**
> Grab a big bottle of water, put it by your desk or wherever you work, or at home in a place where you will see it often. Whenever you take a bite from your lunch box, have a few gulps and aim to finish the bottle by the end of the day.

Caffeine-containing Drinks

Caffeine is one of those good news/bad news things. Many athletes, particularly runners, have used caffeine for years to boost performance. Lots of us enjoy a good 'cup of Java' in the morning as well. Caffeine has been studied for years and every study seems to turn up more findings about its basic physiological effects.

Caffeine is an addictive drug. The way it works in the body is similar to the effects of amphetamines and cocaine, although obviously much milder. It stimulates the brain in much the same way and the more you consume, the more you'll need to get the same effect.

Then you have the good old 'fight or flight' syndrome going on. The body releases adrenaline, your pupils are dilated, your breathing tubes open up, your heart beats faster, blood pressure rises, additional glucose is sent to the bloodstream and your muscles are tight and ready for action. You're ready to go!

Increased blood pressure? Rapid heart beat? Too much glucose in the blood? These are all problematic. People with cardiovascular disease, especially erratic heart beat, should avoid caffeine and those with diabetes should monitor their blood sugar levels carefully if they consume caffeine drinks.

If your health is okay, you don't need to worry about the plain cuppa unless you consume too much. Caffeine in moderate amounts can make you more mentally alert. It's been shown to improve athletic performance because it preserves glycogen (muscle sugar). When muscles run out of glycogen during exertion, this is when pain, cramping and fatigue set in.

So the odd cup of coffee in the morning is fine, but watch out for sugar-laced, creamy lattes, which stack up the calories and saturated fats.

What about energy drinks? First of all, they are usually loaded with sugar. This will blow your weight loss efforts in double-quick time. Secondly, they have extremely high levels of caffeine. And last but not least, they often contain other

'If your health is okay, you don't need to worry about the plain cuppa unless you consume too much'

herbal stimulants such as ginseng and guarana which may or may not sit well with you whether you have medical issues or not. They have a tendency to make you feel jittery because they are sort of super-charged by the caffeine and can have all sorts of short-term immediate effects on blood pressure.

What does Simon say? Save your money and have a cup of Java instead. But remember, when you're following the Lunch Box Diet, you won't have much need for artificial energy because all the good food is going to give you buckets of it. After starting the diet try to break your routine of drinking caffeine drinks so often and see how your energy levels lie, I think you'll be pleasantly surprised!

The key is moderation. You can't drink a pot of coffee and chase caffeine pills with an energy drink. However, a few cups of coffee in the morning or as an afternoon pick me up is perfectly fine if you are otherwise healthy. And when you're following the Lunch Box Diet, you won't have much need for artificial energy because all the good food is going to give you buckets of it.

Teas

Tea is a wonderful source of hydration for your body. Sure, some tea has caffeine but it also contains a unique source of antioxidants. What's more, it will quench your fluid requirements and give you nutrients, yet it won't pack on the pounds in the way that drinking too much juice will. It's like getting an immune system boost capable of fighting off cancer-causing free radicals with no calorific cost. If you want to avoid caffeine there are plenty of herbal teas and de-caff varieties of black tea and green tea. Black tea and green tea both have good levels of antioxidant activity, although they contain a different mix of antioxidants.

Green tea has lots of lovely antioxidants, including an amazing one called Epigallocatechin gallate, or EGCG. EGCG increases metabolism, which is a fabulous benefit for green tea drinkers.

'After starting the diet try to break your routine of drinking caffeine drinks so often and see how your energy levels lie, I think you'll be pleasantly surprised!'

Whatever your cuppa of choice, there's a way to fit the benefits of black tea, green tea and herbal tea into your day. If you normally drink Earl Grey in the morning, try blending it with green tea. Or sample the tasty blends of green and herbal teas that are available now, such as green tea with peppermint, jasmine or lemon. And there is also roobois tea, which is high in antioxidants but contains no caffeine.

Keeping a tasty pot of fresh-brewed tea around is a sure way to fill your fluid requirements. Just brew your own instead of buying sugary, flavoured ones in a bottle.

Fruit Juice

'A juicer is a great addition to any kitchen and you won't believe how much more tasty the real deal is'

Bottled or tinned juice is a bit over-rated in my opinion. A lot of it contains about as much sugar as fizzy drinks and, in some cases, about the same amount of real fruit ... zero! You have to check the labels carefully to find 'juice' that is actually made from real fruits and/or vegetables and not just artificial flavourings. And while orange juice is certainly full of great nutrients, be sure to buy fresh orange juice as opposed to concentrate.

My advice? Make your own juice! A juicer is a great addition to any kitchen and you won't believe how much tastier the real deal is. Combine anything your heart desires instead of relying on the manufacturers to know what tickles your taste buds.

Still, sparingly is the key here. Treat real juice as a serving of food rather than a beverage. You wouldn't suck down a big old smoothie and consider it just a beverage to go with your eggs and toast, would you? The same thought process applies to juice.

Sports Drinks

Nowhere in the non-alcoholic drinks world is marketing more appealing than with the 'sports drinks'. Great shots of rippled athletes sweating and working hard make us all want to go out and buy whatever colourful sports drink it is that these creatures of perfection are drinking. We have to remember, though, that it's the working out (and a load of other things they do or don't do) that makes them healthy, not so much what they drink.

Sports drinks do have merit, mind you. The electrolytes they provide help prevent and fix dehydration more efficiently than water. The problem is that they also contain sugar. So while having a sports drink after a great work out or while out in extreme heat is a wise idea, you can't suck them down one after another during a normal day and think you're going to look like Becks (or Posh for that matter). Use sports drinks only when you're being active.

Milk

There's nothing like a nice cold glass of 'moo juice'! However, easy does it. A little goes a long way. A 250ml glass of skimmed milk contains around 306 grams of calcium (between a quarter and a third of your daily needs) and 80 calories. That may not sound like a lot of calories, but think about the size of glass you normally pour your milk into. Take a measuring jug and measure out 250ml. Most milk lovers would look at this amount in huge disappointment.

The point is, it's quite easy to drink two or even three servings of milk, adding up to 240 calories, which is a good chunk of a meal. So, while I want you all to be getting adequate calcium, remember that calcium is available in other foods as well (see page 132). As we're weight watching here, try to get used to fat-free milk, preferably organic.

Friday Night and it's Time for Fun!

The week is over and you've had a rough one. You want to stop off at the pub for a beverage and diet cola just won't do. But how much will a drink cost you in terms of your dieting efforts?

I'm not going to get preachy here about drinking alcohol. Some folks don't drink at all, some drink a little and some drink too much. I'll leave you to make your own choices, but obviously the less you drink the less you have to burn. There – nuff said! Now, back to FUN!

For the calorie content of some of the most popular alcoholic beverages see the box to your left. Keep in mind the portions: 125ml of wine looks awfully teeny in that giant goblet, and if you like your spirits, remember that they'll cost you more if you've got a generous bartender. That said, I don't want you to worry about counting calories – just get a rough idea of the best choices. Okay?

Wine

One of the best pieces of advice I can give you regarding wine consumption is to become a connoisseur rather than gulping down cheap plonk. Enjoying a glass of really good wine slowly is the key to not overdoing it. If you're spending a bit more you are likely to have fewer glasses, yet you still get to enjoy the wine.

Alternatively, turn your wine into a long, cool drink by spritzing it with zero-calorie fizzy water and lots of ice.

Simon's bite-sized tips

Alcohol Energy Content

Wine 125ml glass 80–100cal

Dessert Wine 125ml glass 120–200cal

Lager 500ml bottle 145cal

Bitter 500ml bottle 160cal

Cider 500ml bottle (dry) 180cal

Spirits (25ml measure) 56 cal

Liqueurs (25ml measure) 60–100+cal

Beer

Due to the no-carb/low-carb craze, a lot of breweries have produced 'low carb' beers. This is merely a marketing ploy and you should look at these beers as 'light' beers. Light beers are the best choice unless, of course, you find them less satisfying and end up drinking more. There are some really great light crisp lagers out there, but if your taste buds are more geared towards heavier beers, you may find them watery.

Have you ever noticed how good a lot of salty, greasy foods taste with beer? Salty foods are complemented by beer so it always seems even more tempting to dig in to the buffet or the bowl of peanuts but these calories can mount up quickly. A serving of nuts of any sort should be no more than a small handful.

Spirits

A measure of spirits has fewer calories than a small glass of wine. This is good news if you like mixing them with diet tonic or cola. Unfortunately, if you prefer fruitier concoctions or non-diet mixers, you're talking about a much higher energy content. Pina Coladas, Mai Tais, Daiquiris and drinks of this nature can have more calories than a Big Mac! You could try mixing a flavoured vodka with a diet soda water to get that fruity flavour, if you're in a bar that has the option. Try these:

- Vanilla vodka mixed with diet orangeade
- Raspberry vodka mixed with diet lemonade
- Strawberry vodka mixed with club soda

Liqueurs

Watch out for the liqueurs. Any more than a tiny 25ml measure will add up quickly. They're meant for sipping and anyone who's had a few too many of these babies knows what a nasty hangover you can expect the next day. Save them for special occasions and make sure you just sip.

Avoiding the Other Pitfalls at the Pub

Make sure you don't drink on an empty stomach. You'll get drunk very easily and may be tempted to gorge yourself on greasy bar snacks. Having a few extra helpings of your lunch box before leaving for the bar will help to line your stomach and control those urges to pig out.

If you get hungry when you're out drinking, choose something light on the bar menu like grilled chicken breast with vegetables or even a cup of soup and half a sandwich. This should do the trick of keeping something in your stomach and helping you to stay away from the tempting deep-fried fare.

Have you started the diet or are you still reading? If you've started, you're probably realising just how much more you're getting out of it than mere weight loss

Chapter 8

Beyond Weight Loss

If you haven't started, get going! I want you to experience all the benefits of optimum nutrition as soon as you can! Once you really get into this diet plan, you're going to realise how much more is improving than just your jean size. You're going to discover a healthier new you!

Energy

Feeling energetic? If you are overweight, chances are one of your chief complaints is lack of energy; however, this can be true even if you aren't overweight but are simply not eating properly. Feeling drained isn't a nice feeling. It's tough to do even the simplest things, let alone work out. No energy for work, no energy for the children, no energy for your partner … To boot, when you are fatigued, it's much more likely that you will succumb to cravings and comfort foods.

Fatigue is a never-ending merry-go-round ride, and it's not any fun at all! Eating badly makes us overweight and/or fatigued and being fatigued makes it difficult to work out and be healthier. Couple that with the weight gain, and you're on a rocky road! And if you seek the happiness a lack of energy is depriving you of in a bag of crisps or a box of chocolates, it all goes further downhill.

The fantastic foods you will be eating on the Lunch Box Diet will provide you with optimum energy and nutrition. What you are doing is making your body a lean fighting machine. Everything is working correctly, functioning properly and running at optimum efficiency and speed. All that damage you've done to your body over the years by not treating your body well will slowly disappear as you change your eating habits.

I can't emphasise enough what a gift it is to have energy! I never knew what I was missing before I started eating properly and working out. You're going to be surprised at how fantastic you feel. And more energy will definitely lead you to the gym, perhaps mine. What's more, it will also make you more attractive and could even help you find a new lover. Exciting, eh?

'If you haven't started, get going! I want you to experience all the benefits of optimum nutrition as soon as you can!'

Hair, Skin and Nails

I've been told by many women that it's the accessories that make an outfit work. Just as a great pair of shoes or a stunning piece of jewellery will accentuate an outfit, the health of your built-in accessories (hair, skin and nails) will accentuate your body. Just as a tattered scarf can ruin the look of a beautiful dress, so will dull skin and raggedy hair –and it's the same for us guys.

When we're little kids, we've got it made. It doesn't matter what you do to children's hair, it still grows beautifully with a sheen and brilliance. So what happens? As we get older, our body's ability to regenerate itself on a cellular level decreases. When cells can't regenerate as quickly or repair themselves, we find that our hair grows more poorly, our skin doesn't look so hot, our nails split and we are more susceptible to any number of illnesses.

Why bother, then? If it's going to happen to us all, just let nature take its course. Wrong! You see, how soon and at what pace all this occurs is up to us. We can't control all the toxins out there that cause cellular damage, but we can help our body to defend itself against them. We can help our cells regenerate themselves at optimum level if we give them the proper tools. What if I told you to build a house and handed you wood and nails but no hammer? It's the same for the cells.

Nearly every function in our body relies on the food we consume. When you eat junk instead of healthy foods, your body isn't getting everything it needs to perform daily functions, yet it still has to do them. Certain functions hold higher priority, such as breathing and your heart beating.

The condition of hair, skin and nails is a good indication of overall health. Women tend to cover up yellow, brittle nails by using polish. The problem is that this out-of-sight/out-of-mind theory will only serve to hide more serious issues resulting from nutritional deficiencies.

So what gets put on the back burner? You guessed it: non-essentials like a beautiful head of hair, glowing skin and strong, healthy nails.

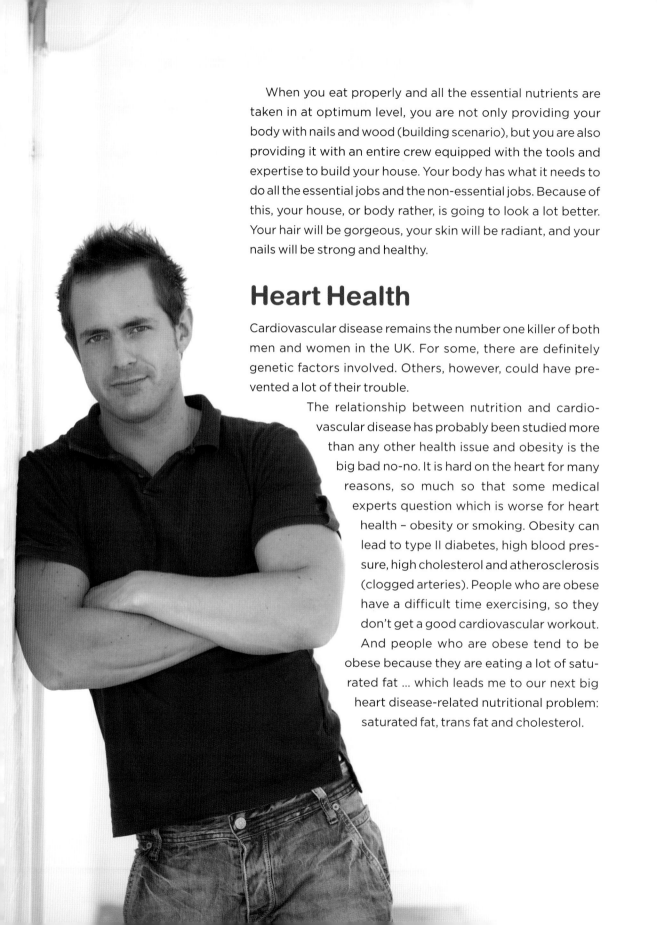

When you eat properly and all the essential nutrients are taken in at optimum level, you are not only providing your body with nails and wood (building scenario), but you are also providing it with an entire crew equipped with the tools and expertise to build your house. Your body has what it needs to do all the essential jobs and the non-essential jobs. Because of this, your house, or body rather, is going to look a lot better. Your hair will be gorgeous, your skin will be radiant, and your nails will be strong and healthy.

Heart Health

Cardiovascular disease remains the number one killer of both men and women in the UK. For some, there are definitely genetic factors involved. Others, however, could have prevented a lot of their trouble.

The relationship between nutrition and cardiovascular disease has probably been studied more than any other health issue and obesity is the big bad no-no. It is hard on the heart for many reasons, so much so that some medical experts question which is worse for heart health – obesity or smoking. Obesity can lead to type II diabetes, high blood pressure, high cholesterol and atherosclerosis (clogged arteries). People who are obese have a difficult time exercising, so they don't get a good cardiovascular workout. And people who are obese tend to be obese because they are eating a lot of saturated fat ... which leads me to our next big heart disease-related nutritional problem: saturated fat, trans fat and cholesterol.

Fats and Cholesterol

Saturated fats and trans fats have been related to an increased risk of heart disease because of their effect on blood cholesterol levels. There are two main kinds of cholesterol – one which is bad for you, known as LDL, and one that is good, known as HDL. Diets high in saturated fat and trans fat tend to raise LDL cholesterol, the bad guy. Saturated fat is present in high amounts in fatty meats, greasy fast foods and butter-rich cooking, which is exactly why I advocate lean meat choices for protein. Trans fats are scientifically altered fats that are found in deep fried fast foods and some snack foods and biscuits.

When we fuel our bodies with poor protein choices, we miss out on the benefits of the good fats in leaner choices such as fish and nuts. Fish, nuts and even the good old egg have healthy polyunsaturated fats called omega-3 and omega-6. These fats work to lower LDL (bad) and raise HDL (good). Contrary to the previous belief that eggs had a negative effect on cholesterol, later research and clarification has put the egg back on the good guy list.

When LDL levels are high, cholesterol is deposited on the walls of the arteries. This forms plaques that make it harder for the blood to circulate and is known as arteriosclerosis. Conversely, HDL is capable of taking away the extra cholesterol and transporting it to the liver from where it is excreted. Not only that, but HDL can also remove cholesterol that is already attached to the artery walls.

Adequate vitamin and mineral intake is also imperative for good cardiovascular health. All those vegetables you consume in your lunch box do a lot of good for your heart. Those antioxidants we discussed earlier help to make all the organs work more efficiently and some of them can help to clear excess cholesterol.

The heart is a muscle and, like all muscles, it benefits from exercise. We'll be looking at heart-healthy exercises later on in this chapter.

Bone Health

The Lunch Box Diet doesn't include many dairy products. I know what you're thinking: 'I'm supposed to drink milk to prevent bone loss and osteoporosis, and this berk is trying to make me cut down on it.' This is both false and true. Repeat after me: 'It is not necessary to consume large quantities of dairy products in order to reduce bone loss or prevent osteoporosis.' Sure, you need adequate calcium, but that is abundant in many of the foods you consume in the Lunch Box Diet.

Bone breaks itself down and rebuilds itself all day long. It's called remodelling. Up until the age of 30, our bones naturally keep up with all the building up and breaking down. After 30, regardless of what you did before or are doing now, it's the natural tendency of bone not to be able to keep up on the rebuilding end. But all hope is not lost.

What you do up until the age of 30 dictates quite a bit what will happen to your body afterwards. If you have nutritionally supported your bones, exercised and abstained from smoking and you continue to do so, you're going to be in pretty good shape in terms of overall bone health. It's like putting money in the bank to survive tougher times ahead. If you haven't made enough deposits in the bone bank, you're going to have to work even harder. Here's how.

Obesity is a key factor in bone health. Excess weight places a lot of strain and wear and tear on the skeleton. Joints are especially affected by obesity and this can lead to debilitating problems such as knee trouble. So achieving and maintaining a healthy body weight is key in bone health.

As I've said, adequate calcium is important but you don't need to guzzle a gallon of milk. There is a lot of calcium in dark leafy greens such as kale and collard greens. As a matter of fact, one cup of collard greens contains more calcium than one cup of skimmed milk. Dried beans and legumes also contain calcium. Oranges have a bit, as do almonds. And salmon! Salmon is a wonderful source of calcium. Check out the box on the left to compare calcium amounts. However, you should know that the

Simon's bite-sized tips

Calcium Sources

Dairy
Fat-free milk, 250ml 306 mg
Yoghurt, plain, 1 cup 415 mg
Cottage cheese, 1 cup 138 mg

Plant Sources
Collards, 1 cup steamed 357 mg
Spinach, 1 cup steamed 291 mg
Black-eyed peas, 1 cup cooked 211 mg
Green peas, 1 cup 94 mg
A medium orange 72 mg
Almonds, 24 70 mg

Animal Sources
Tinned Salmon, 80g 181 mg

Vitamin D is also important for bone health because when calcium is low in the blood, the body changes vitamin D into its active form, which increases calcium absorption and minimises its excretion.

oxalic acid in spinach and chard means that the calcium is a little less well absorbed than calcium from other sources.

How are you getting vitamin D in the Lunch Box Diet? Salmon, tuna and eggs. You can also look for soya products that are fortified with vitamin D, or make a smoothie in the morning with skimmed milk or yoghurt, and you probably have a great deal of your vitamin D requirements covered. And don't forget that sunlight is an important source of vitamin D.

Vitamin K is another big one. It helps osteocalcin, a bone matrix protein, to function properly. Vitamin K is easy to get in the Lunch Box Diet because it is found in spinach, collards, broccoli, and other dark leafy greens.

Phosphorus is important in maintaining bone strength and it is present in beans, soya, nuts and wholegrains. Magnesium is also vital and it's found in many fruits, veggies, wholegrains, red meat, poultry and dairy.

Again, exercise is important in maintaining bone health. Studies show that women who exercise keep their bones strong and have a reduced incidence of hip fractures and osteoporosis. Isn't it worth it for that alone?

'Sure, you need adequate calcium, but that is abundant in many of the foods you consume in the Lunch Box Diet'

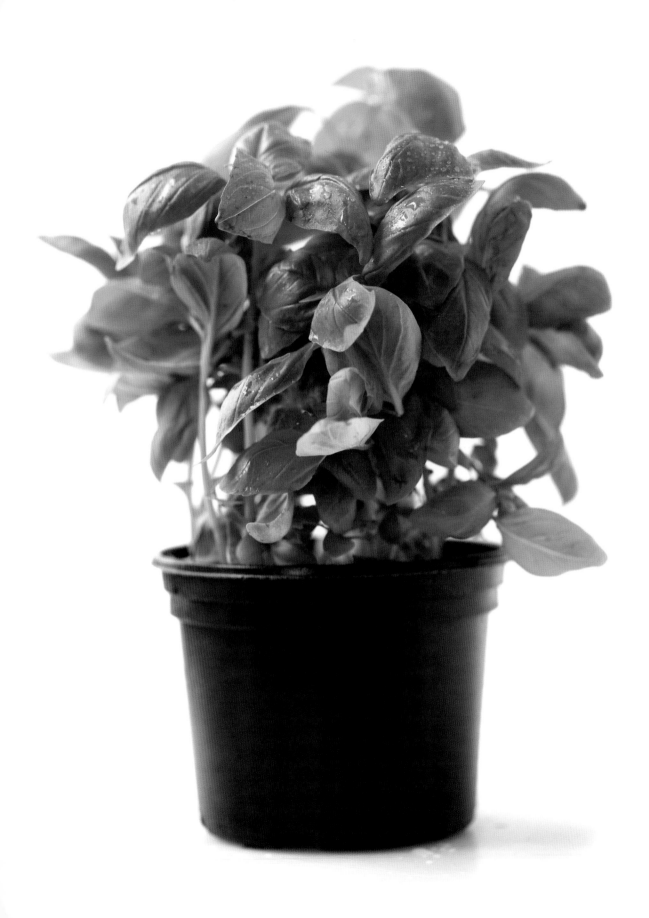

Hormonal Balance

Hormones control virtually every activity. Without getting too technical, you should understand that the basic building blocks of hormones are all those vitamins, minerals and proteins that I keep telling you about. So, if you're not eating properly and your body is consistently missing out on these things, your hormones aren't going to function properly.

Thyroid problems can upset your hormonal balance. When the thyroid becomes too slow (hypo) or too fast (hyper), it does all sorts of horrendous things to the body. There can be uncontrollable weight gain or weight loss, fatigue and hair loss. Calcium is stripped from the body so bones can become fragile and dental health deteriorates. Sleep becomes difficult. Night sweats, shaky hands and bulging eyes are part of the condition. Worst of all, your heart is affected and ultimately, if they continue untreated, thyroid problems can cause irreversible damage to your heart. As with any symptoms that are disrupting your life and causing you worry, you should definitely seek the advice of a physician. A simple blood test is performed to determine the status of your thyroid.

Hormonal imbalance causes menstrual problems for women. Some fluctuation during the menstrual cycle is normal, crucial and expected. The hormones fluctuating are, after all, what regulates the cycle. However, many, many women can experience extreme mood swings, irritability, inability to concentrate, very heavy bleeding and severe pain.

Good nutrition can help to prevent extreme hormone imbalances and to correct them once they have appeared. All those veggies that are in the lunch box provide the body with the proper building blocks for hormones. There are even some that may have a direct effect on women's hormones, such as the sweet potato. Avoiding alcohol and caffeine can help and exercising can really be beneficial. Whenever one of my female clients comes in and warns me that she's 'in a mood', I direct her to the punch bag! It seems to help.

Cancer Prevention

Cancer is a frightening, frightening word. Many people can't even say it out loud, as if the mere utterance will bring that terrible disease into their lives.

A lot of whether or not we'll end up with cancer has to do with our genes – something we didn't have much choice about. It also has to do with our environment, which we're not completely in control of. But it's not all bad news!

Scientists are finding out new things about cancer all the time. Though the Lunch Box Diet wasn't created to prevent cancer, it just so happens that it follows a lot of cancer-prevention advice that the scientists are giving us. All those vitamins, especially the antioxidants, have been shown to decrease the risk of developing certain cancers. Eating a diet with adequate amounts of fibre has been shown to decrease the risk of bowel cancer. Eating a diet low in saturated fat has been shown to reduce the risk of developing many cancers. Maintaining a healthy body weight helps to prevent many different types of cancer, including breast cancer.

The Lunch Box Diet advocates fresh and organic. When we eat fresh foods, we replace all those preservatives and artificial additives that in high quantities may be cancer-causing; eating organic whenever possible helps to keep some nasty chemicals out of your diet.

And here's the best part. Scientists keep finding out great things about the benefits of the different vitamins found in different vegetables, so you really can't go wrong if you're consuming a wide variety of veg. Make sure you get each and every one of those vitamins and minerals they're talking about!

All in all, I just wanted you to know how much more you're getting out of this diet than merely weight loss – which is a big one all on its own. You truly are changing your life for the better. Not only will you be slim and look fabulous in those skinny jeans or tight T-shirt, but your skin and hair will be gorgeous as well. Most importantly, you will be doing everything you can to prevent terrible diseases that would be devastating to you and your loved ones.

Your Exercise

Exercise is my first love when it comes to health and fitness and I know it will make you feel more alive, confident and sexier than ever. I appreciate that it can take a few sessions to get going but once that snowball starts rolling, it will never stop and you'll look back and think, 'Why has it taken me this long?'

One problem is that too many people go to gyms without an exercise plan and expect to know what they're doing – but let me ask you, would you have driven a car for the first time without taking driving lessons? No! So we shouldn't really expect to know what we're doing when we start exercising. You need advice on the intensity, the amount of repetitions when performing weights, and many other things.

If you've tried going to the gym but came out after a few months feeling disillusioned and looking the same as when you went in, it could be for one of these reasons:

- You hardly worked up a sweat, yet used the fact you had exercised as an excuse to have pie and chips for dinner.
- You went from one machine to the other for five or ten minutes on each, did exactly the same for six weeks and are still paying the gym membership a year later.
- You weren't aware of how important it was to set goals and implement a weight-training programme.
- There was help around but you were too afraid to ask the trainer, book in for a programme and really feel the benefits.
- Sweating it out in the steam room seemed like the best use of your membership, but then you found out that any weight you lost was water!

Hiring a personal trainer is my firm advice for anyone starting out at the gym (and it's not just because I am one). Even a couple of sessions will help you to work out an effective programme and set goals that will keep you motivated.

Finding Time for Working Out

If one of my newer clients doesn't show up for a session, they get punished severely with extra crunches! Here are some suggestions to get you going.

- Free up your schedule and make time for exercise. It will give you buckets of energy that will help you get more done in less time.
- When you have a spare five minutes, grab a skipping rope and see how many jumps you can get in.
- Instead of the usual dinner and cinema, why not go dancing? Believe me, you can really burn up some calories!
- Instead of meeting friends at the usual café or restaurant, suggest that you meet for a fun exercise class or tennis.
- Get involved in a team sport. There are a lot of options in most clubs or community centres.

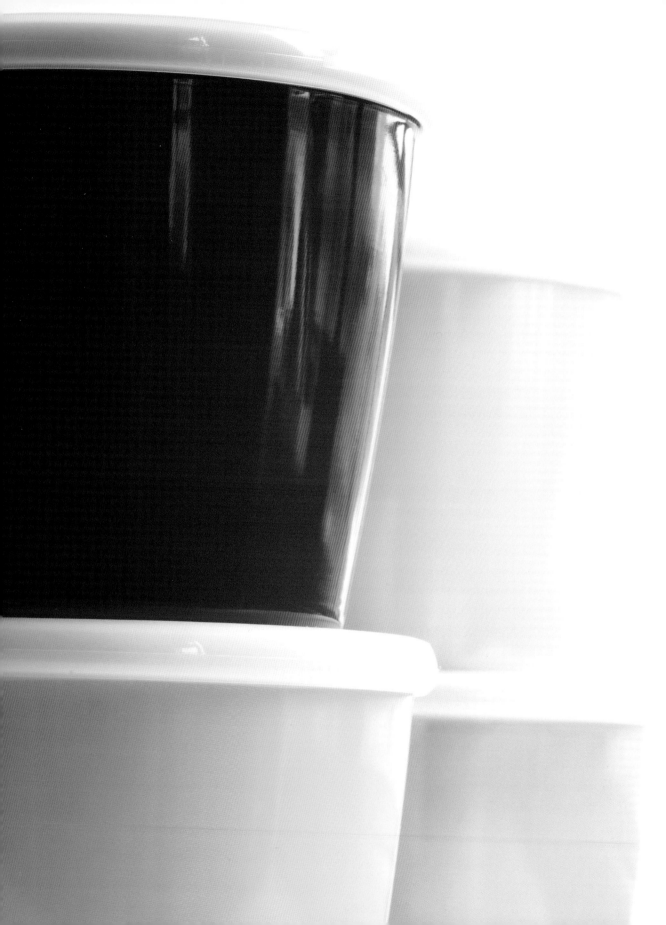

It is possible to lose weight without exercising and I'm not telling you that you need to live in the gym or become a marathon runner to achieve your ideal body weight, but there are loads of reasons to delve into the wonderful world of exercise. Here are just a few:

- Cardiovascular health – Study after study shows that people who exercise regularly are far less likely to succumb to cardiovascular disease. Exercise lowers blood pressure and decreases cholesterol levels. Remember that your heart is a muscle and working it through aerobic exercise makes it stronger.
- Bone health – Studies show that exercise is almost of equal importance to nutrition in maintaining bone density and strengthening the muscle surrounding the bone.
- Energy – Work out for one week along with eating properly via all you've learned thus far and I guarantee you the energy you will have will be phenomenal – like a kid when they first arrive at Disneyland!
- Stress – There's nothing like a good work out to reduce stress. How often do you eat because you're stressed out? If you took this stressful moment and ran it off on the treadmill or abused a punching bag for even 15 minutes, you'd be doing your mind a world of good (and your significant other for that matter).
- Thin or sexy? – Lose all the weight you want but without toning and firming exercises, that bikini may as well stay on the rail at the store. Maybe you couldn't give a hoot about six-pack abs and a tight bum, but I'm betting most of you want to look just as sexy naked as you do in a savvy black business suit. You won't believe how easy it is to take your weight loss one step further and sculpt your body into a gorgeous work of art!

I'm going to give you some basic ideas that will help get you going whether you have an unused gym membership card in your wallet or a dusty treadmill that's got lost under a pile of clothes.

Affordable Equipment for Home

- Stability ball
- Flex bands
- Dumbbells for beginners (3, 4, 5 kilos for women, 8, 10, 12 for men)
- Yoga mat, blocks and strap
- Medicine balls (2, 3, 4 kilos)
- Skipping rope
- Step
- Boxing gloves and hitting pads (great with two people)

Cardio

Cardio is a good way to burn off extra weight. It's also important for good cardiovascular health. You really can't go wrong with cardio because it does a lot of things for your body in even its simplest form. Let's go over your options.

Interval Training

A great way of burning fat and creating more of a hormonal response in the body is to work for short periods at a high intensity, and I'd really advise this if you get bored easily during exercise. Instead of jogging for 30 minutes you could try performing your cardio exercise for short bursts and then resting. Increase the intensity over time, either by increasing the work time or reducing the rest time. This could also be applied to speed walking if you're a beginner. Overall you'd still be working for 30 minutes, just in a different way. You can apply this principle to any exercise: use a stop watch and observe those rest times.

Machines at the Gym

There are a number of cardio options available at most clubs. Treadmills are fantastic and fairly easy to operate. If you're curious about the other stranger-looking machines, grab a trainer and he or she will be glad to show you exactly how to use them. Cross-trainers are very popular these days, but be sure to work up a sweat. Fixed cycling machines, Stairmasters and Steppers are great for slicing off the fat, but again you need to work hard for the best results.

Swimming

Swimming is an excellent cardio exercise that is extremely gentle on the body. It's good for people who have joint problems that make running or walking difficult and works a bunch muscle groups that aren't used as much for we land-dwellers. Take a friend and have races to stop it getting tedious doing length after length. If you can't swim, now's the time to learn.

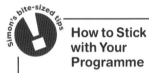

Simon's bite-sized tips

How to Stick with Your Programme

- Change your routine at least monthly
- Listen to upbeat music
- Wear an outfit you feel good in
- Get your friends involved
- Try a new sport
- Hire a trainer for continuous motivation
- Work beyond your comfort zone and feel the buzz afterwards
- Try boxing; it's great for women and men and decreases stress like nothing else!

Walking/Jogging/Running

Walking, jogging or running outdoors definitely has its advantages – not least the ever-changing scenery, which a gym can't offer. Start the day with a run in the morning or a brisk walk to work. Lunch breaks can be a good time to exercise because on the Lunch Box Diet you don't need long to eat a meal. Take a few bites, grab a water bottle and go for a quick power walk. You'll come back to the office feeling super fresh and energetic. Night-time walks can be the perfect way to de-stress after a long day. After dinner has settled, put on those running shoes, crank up the tunes and hit the pavement.

Buy yourself a good pair of running or walking shoes because running or walking on pavements can be quite hard on the joints. Stretching properly and adding strength training to your routine can help with this, but good shoes are a must!

Strength Training

Training with weights not only improves joint health and aids in injury prevention (when done properly), but it also adds that sexy factor to your weight-loss programme. It's like this: losing weight will get those heads turning when you walk by, but firming, toning and building muscle will cause those head turns to become fast-paced neck injuries! The more muscle in the body, the less room for fat. Muscle speeds up metabolism and by now you know how important that is. All my clients work with weights and as a result they have a superior body shape and burn calories even after our sessions have ended. Gals, if you want to look fabulous in a bikini and, guys, if you want to make women drool over your lean stomach and toned pecs, pay attention!

To increase muscle and tone up you can use weights or your own body as resistance. You should work on each exercise until your muscle gets tired. If working to the correct intensity you may well feel soreness for a couple of days after. This is usual – it's the body repairing itself after your muscle tissue has been slightly broken down, so don't be worried.

Calorie Burn

Simon's bite-sized tips

Calories burned per half hour

Walking at 4 mph
185 calories

Running at 6 mph
258 calories

Elliptical machine
350-400 calories

Skipping rope
(easy) 309 calories
(intense) 338 calories

Kickboxing 330 calories

Weight training 176 calories

Yoga 116 calories

Cycling at 5.5 mph
122 calories

Dancing (intense)
256 calories

Swimming (slow crawl)
244 calories

Yoga

When practised properly, yoga is gentle on the body yet able to strengthen and tone muscles you didn't even know you had. There are two basic approaches: traditional yoga that is based on original Hindu yoga practices and Westernised practice that involves less of the spiritual aspect. Both are wonderful – it's really just a matter of personal preference or style.

Yoga is practised at various levels from beginner right on up to advanced. You focus on breathing, meditation, strength, flexibility and, in power yoga, calorie burning. Classes are led by teachers, who will help if you have trouble understanding a pose. There are also some very good DVDs if you want to do it yourself at home. Start with one aimed at beginners and work your way up.

Pilates

Pilates was originally developed to help people rehabilitating from injury after World War One and has now become an extremely successful and popular form of exercise. One of the key principles is that you build strong core muscles in your stomach, bum, pelvis and thighs, which keeps your posture straight and tall and protects your back – and it's great for flattening your stomach! You can practise mat exercises at home, but in the Pilates studio they have big, spring-loaded machines known as reformers where you do muscle-strengthening resistance exercises safely, supervised by instructors.

Martial Arts

Martial arts are a great way to burn a ton of calories, build muscle strength and learn self-defence as well. There are many, many forms from kickboxing to Tae-Kwon-Do and all offer the same benefits. For lighter intensity, try T'ai Chi. Kickboxing usually starts out pretty basic and most can handle it, but it can also move into the intense level. Some of the heavier forms of martial arts include Jiu-Jitsu, Brazilian Jiu-Jitsu and Muay Thai.

Lots of gyms and martial arts studios offer introductory classes, which are definitely worth trying. If you want to work from home, there are some good DVDs that will help.

Simon's bite-sized tips

Increasing Calorie Burn via Everyday Routines

- Turn up the tunes. High-energy music while you're doing everyday activities, from showering to washing the dishes, will get you moving and improve your mood as well.
- You've heard the tip about taking the stairs instead of the lift. Push it to the next level and take that flight of steps twice!
- If you have a car, wash it yourself instead of running it through the automated carwash.
- If you have a lawn to mow, do yourself and the planet a favour and purchase a manual lawnmower. They are fantastic for burning calories as they are a lot tougher to push.

Exercise and Your Kids

Children today live in a world of screens: television, game consoles, computers, handheld games. No generation before these guys have had so many options that all have one thing in common: sitting on their bums!

As a former gamer myself (and a chubbier fellow at that time) I can sympathise. Games are a lot of fun. Computers are not only fun but educational as well and the TV isn't bad if they are guided towards the more informative programmes and away from cartoons. It's tough! So many choices, so little time.

First of all, if you can afford to make the switch, I highly recommend purchasing a Wii. These have sports and fitness games that involve standing, moving and waving a wand around in front of the screen, so at least they'll get your child up and about. Perhaps you should have them switch arms occasionally, though. I've had clients come in with painful arm muscles caused by playing on their child's Wii!

You need to set limits about screen time. Perhaps they could even earn it by performing exercises for you. For example, 100 star jumps for 30 minutes of computer time or run around the house 10 times for a cartoon break.

Getting children to enjoy exercise is key. You have to be creative and tune in to what your child enjoys. Do they like music? Pump up the tunes and do some dancing together. They will probably make fun of your moves but that's par for the course as a parent.

With the Lunch Box Diet you are free to put together your own combinations and then eat your normal breakfast and evening meal – but if you're looking for a plan to follow then I've come up with a 28-day solution

Chapter 9

Your 28-Day Plan

If you can't commit to 28 days, start with two or three. Don't worry if the breakfast and evening meal suggestions don't suit your family life – just relax and eat what you would normally. You should feel less hungry after eating from your lunch box throughout the day so just eat until you're satisfied.

In preparation for your first week on the Lunch Box Diet, set off to the supermarket or your local grocers and get filling those baskets full of colourful ingredients. Stock your cupboards now with lots of herbs and other dressings from group C and get rid of the rubbish so you're not tempted to pick on unhealthy foods. You don't have to include the exercise days but they're advisable for optimum results.

The day before you start, I want you to weigh yourself and take a waist measurement. You won't do this again until the end of the four weeks. This is because weight fluctuates day in day out, so relax, take it now but resist temptation to check it constantly and you will thank me at the end of week four!

There are a couple of other motivational tips you can try. It's a good idea to tell friends and family what you are doing so that they can support and encourage you. You might find it helpful to write messages to yourself and stick them up around the house – especially in the kitchen. And perhaps you have some outfit that is too tight at the moment; try it on the night before you diet and then don't try it again until the end of the four weeks when, with any luck, it will fit!

My Info	
Weight:	
Waist measurement:	
How I feel about my current weight:	
How I feel about life right now:	
My current energy levels:	

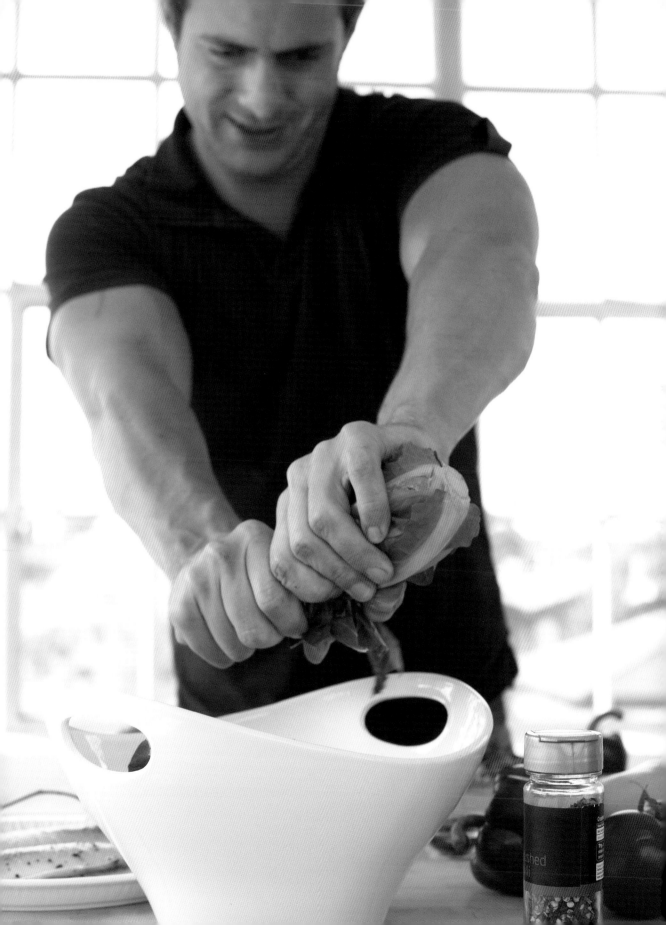

Week 1

Get your foods ready for day one. I've suggested you start on a Monday but it could be any other day. Notice when you can use leftovers from dinner the night before in your lunch box – for example, if you make extra grilled chicken on day one, you can use it for lunch on day two. Get a big bottle of water to put by your desk and off you go!

Day 1 – Monday

Breakfast: 2 poached eggs, 1 slice wholewheat toast (no butter), fresh herbs and freshly ground black pepper

Lunch box: Legume I Presume? (see page 207)

Evening meal: Grilled chicken and roast vegetables

Exercise: 30-minute fitness session

Day 2 – Tuesday

Breakfast: Fibre-based cereal and fresh fruit

Lunch box: Chicken Tango (see page 200)

Evening meal: Grilled fish with fresh herbs and mixed vegetables

Exercise: Rest day

Day 3 – Wednesday

Breakfast: Natural yoghurt with fresh fruit and whole oats

Lunch box: Eggstrordinaire (see page 198)

Evening meal: Home-made curry (your choice) served with brown rice

Exercise: Weight-training session

Day 4 – Thursday

Breakfast: Scrambled eggs (2), 1 slice wholewheat toast, fresh herbs and freshly ground black pepper
Lunch box: Sassy Shrimp (see page 179)
Evening meal: Lean steak, sweet potato and green vegetables
Exercise: Rest day

Day 5 – Friday

Breakfast: Fibre-based cereal and fresh fruit
Lunch box: Beef Bonanza (see page 186)
Evening meal: Roast chicken, vegetables and oven chips
Exercise: 30-minute fitness session

Day 6 – Saturday

Breakfast: Natural yoghurt served with mixed nuts and fruit
Lunch box: Slippery Sardine (see page 164)
Evening meal: Pork, vegetables and a tomato-based sauce
Exercise: Rest day

Day 7 – Sunday

Breakfast: Fresh fruit salad
Lunch: Sunday roast lamb (lean meat and vegetables, but no roast potatoes)
Evening meal: Grilled fish, vegetables
Exercise: Weight-training session

Week 2

Your energy levels should be up, you'll
be feeling less hungry at dinner time and
hopefully you're beginning to see how
eating little and often can have a major
effect on your life. Lost that three o'clock
slump? Well done! What about the exercise?
Feeling great from increasing your heart
rate? The effects of the diet will play on
your attitude towards fitness, so stick
with it and keep smiling!

Day 8 – Monday

Breakfast: Baked beans on 1 slice wholewheat toast with
Worcester sauce, fresh herbs and a sprinkle of grated
cheese on top (to make this healthier, add tinned beans
to your own homemade tomato sauce – see page 85)

Lunch box: Little Lamb (see page 189)

Evening meal: Home-made soup with chicken chunks

Exercise: 45-minute fitness session

Day 9 – Tuesday

Breakfast: Fibre or oat-based cereal with fresh fruit

Lunch box: Beany Berry (see page 211)

Evening meal: Fillet of fish and steamed vegetables

Exercise: Rest day

Day 10 – Wednesday

Breakfast: 2 poached eggs on 1 slice wholewheat toast
with herbs and black pepper

Lunch box: Trendy Tuna (see page 168)

Evening meal: Homemade beef stew

Exercise: Weight-training session

Day 11 – Thursday

Breakfast: Natural yoghurt with fresh fruit and whole oats
Lunch box: Steamy Sea (see page 176)
Evening meal: Stir fry with chicken and oriental vegetables
Exercise: Rest day

Day 12 – Friday

Breakfast: Fibre or oat-based cereal with fresh fruit
Lunch box: Crab Attack (see page 180)
Evening meal: Half a homemade pizza (see page 110)
Exercise: 45-minute fitness session

Day 13 – Saturday

Breakfast: Baked beans on 1 slice wholewheat toast with Worcester sauce, fresh herbs and a sprinkle of grated cheese on top (as on Monday, make your own baked beans)
Lunch box: Spicy Scrambler (see page 204)
Evening meal: Steak, sweet potato mash and some gravy
Exercise: Rest day

Day 14 – Sunday

Breakfast: Fresh fruit salad
Lunch: Sunday roast beef (lean meat and vegetables, but no roast potatoes or Yorkshire puds!)
Evening meal: Grilled fish, vegetables
Exercise: Weight-training session

Week 3

Not so hard is it? Grazing **throughout the** day, a bit of exercise **and I bet you're feeling fantastic. Started thinking about those new** clothes **yet?** Your tummy **should be less bloated by now. Try reducing the** quantities **in your** lunch box **this week and see if it still lasts you through the day.**

Day 15 – Monday

Breakfast: Wholemeal bagel, 2 scrambled eggs, chopped tomatoes and black pepper

Lunch box: Fruity Tofuti (see page 208)

Evening meal: Steamed swordfish with vegetables and wild rice

Exercise: 1-hour fitness session

Day 16 – Tuesday

Breakfast: Fibre or oat-based cereal with fresh fruit

Lunch box: Mighty Sword (see page 167)

Evening meal: Homemade stew with lamb and vegetables

Exercise: Rest day

Day 17 – Wednesday

Breakfast: Natural yoghurt with fresh fruit and mixed nuts

Lunch box: Razzle Dazzle (see page 196)

Evening meal: Grilled fish, vegetables and couscous

Exercise: Weight-training session

Day 18 – Thursday

Breakfast: Baked beans on 1 slice wholewheat toast with Worcester sauce, fresh herbs and a sprinkle of grated cheese on top (make your own tomato sauce for the beans – see page 85)
Lunch box: Bashful Pork (see page 190)
Evening meal: Homemade curry with chicken
Exercise: Rest day

Day 19 – Friday

Breakfast: Wholemeal bagel, 2 scrambled eggs, chopped tomatoes and black pepper
Lunch box: Lip-Smackin' Mack (see page 170)
Evening meal: Beef wrap (see page 112)
Exercise: 1-hour fitness session

Day 20 – Saturday

Breakfast: Fibre or oat-based cereal with fresh fruit
Lunch box: Hot Elegant Beef (see page 185)
Evening meal: Homemade roasted vegetable lasagne (easy on the cheese)
Exercise: Rest day

Day 21 – Sunday

Breakfast: Fresh fruit salad
Lunch: Sunday roast pork (lean meat and vegetables, but no roast potatoes or crackling!)
Evening meal: Grilled fish, vegetables
Exercise: Weight-training session

Week 4

By this stage you should have worked out how much you need in your lunch box to keep you satisfied until your evening meal. I hope you're going to stick with this kind of routine week in week out. Sure, have a few treats and nights out but keep them occasional. Keep going and good luck!

Day 22 – Monday

Breakfast: Baked beans on 1 slice wholewheat toast with Worcester sauce, fresh herbs and a sprinkle of grated cheese (make your own tomato sauce for the beans)
Lunch box: Lean Bellied Pork (see page 192)
Evening meal: Home-made fish stew with tomato-based sauce
Exercise: 1-hour fitness session

Day 23 – Tuesday

Breakfast: Natural yoghurt with fresh fruits and mixed nuts
Lunch box: Sweet and Sour Fish (see page 173)
Evening meal: Home-made soup with chicken chunks
Exercise: Rest day

Day 24 – Wednesday

Breakfast: 2 poached eggs on 1 slice wholewheat toast, topped with fresh herbs and black pepper
Lunch box: Market Ham (see page 195)
Evening meal: Salmon steak baked in a parcel with lemon juice and served with fresh vegetables
Exercise: Weight-training session

Day 25 – Thursday

Breakfast: Fibre-based cereal and fresh fruit

Lunch box: Sexy Salmon (see page 174)

Evening meal: Oven-baked turkey steak with tomato sauce and vegetables

Exercise: Rest day

Day 26 – Friday

Breakfast: Baked beans on 1 slice wholewheat toast with Worcester sauce, fresh herbs and a sprinkle of grated cheese (make your own tomato sauce for the beans)

Lunch box: Trim Turkey (see page 198)

Evening meal: Homemade lamb stew with steamed vegetables

Exercise: 1-hour fitness session

Day 27 – Saturday

Breakfast: Natural yoghurt with fresh fruits and mixed nuts

Lunch box: Sweet Prawn (see page 183)

Evening meal: Spicy beef stir-fry served with quinoa

Exercise: Rest Day

Day 28 – Sunday

Breakfast: Fresh fruit salad

Lunch: Sunday roast pork (lean meat and vegetables, but no roast potatoes or crackling!)

Evening meal: Grilled fish, vegetables

Exercise: Weight-training session

Okay, now you've completed your four weeks it's time to take those vital measurements again. Chances are you've done really well, so after filling this in, cut it out and stick it up on display somewhere that will keep you motivated. If you ever steer off course, you can look back and see how much the Lunch Box Diet changed your life. There will be hurdles along the way, but in just four weeks your body will have changed a great deal as the nutrients it has received via all-natural food enhance your body functions and energy levels. Congratulations!

Re-evaluation: My Info	
Weight:	
Waist measurement:	
How I feel about my current weight:	
How I feel about life right now:	
My current energy levels:	

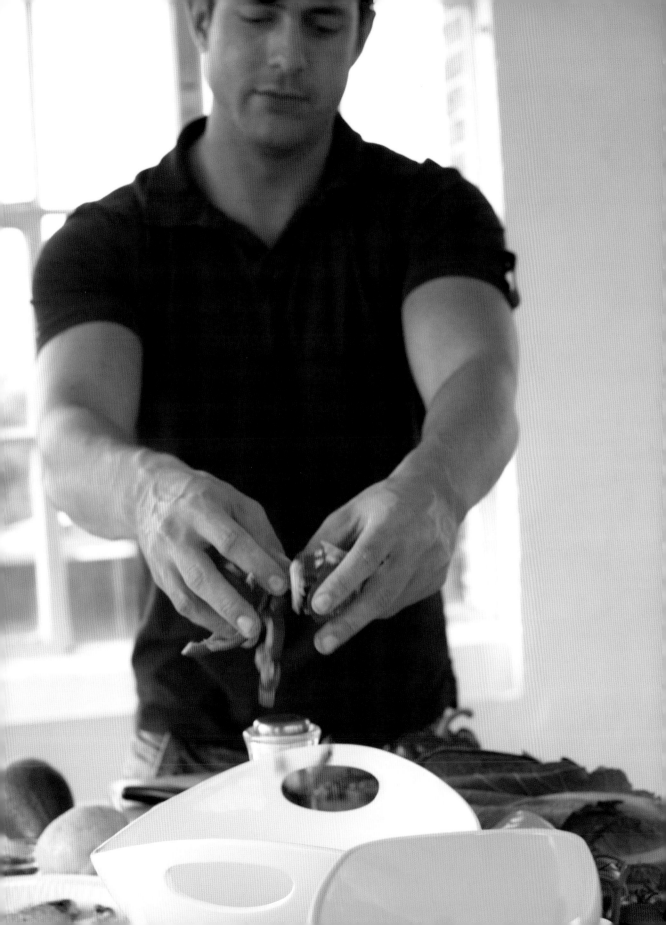

Here are some of my favourite recipes to get you started. Don't be afraid to swap things around if your taste buds tell you to do so!

Chapter 10
Simon's Lunch Box Diet Recipes

Simon's bite-sized tips

Active Carbs

If you have really high energy levels, you can also add an active carb option to any of the recipes. I have suggested an active carb for each recipe, but you can always choose another active carb from the list (see page 40) if you prefer. The quantities will vary according to your activity levels, but the active carb should make up 10–30% of your box (30% for very high activity levels). You should also add an active carb if you suffer from diabetes.

Portion Sizes

Poultry/Beef/Pork (except for ham): 80 grams/deck of cards

Fish: 100 grams (slightly larger than a deck of cards)

Shellfish: 100 grams (lump or good handful of crab/lobster; 3–5 large prawns, depending on size; 12–15 or more of teeny salad shrimps)

Ham: 30 grams

Eggs: 1 or 2 is acceptable

Tofu/Legumes: ½ cup

When preparing your boxes, keep it as simple as possible. Cook meats the night before along with your evening meal, buy bags of pre-cut, pre-washed veggies. Or prepare your vegetables when you get them back from the supermarket and store them in freezer bags in your fridge.

The quantities listed in the recipes in this chapter can be adjusted according to the size of your box and the amount you find you need to get you through the day. If you have an active life and need a bit more, just add more.

Remember that a serving of protein is about the size of a deck of cards unless otherwise noted in the recipes. You can prepare the protein any way you like so long as you aren't adding lots of oils, butter or other fatty flavouring. When you use a deli meat, just pull some out of the package and set it in a little pile on the counter until you get roughly that deck of cards size.

I've tended to go with fresh fish in these recipes, but you can also use tinned fish. Where possible, try using fish that has been tinned in spring water. And if you're using frozen meat or fish, make sure you defrost it properly first. Plant protein sources such as legumes and tofu are around ½ cup per serving. Measure this at first and you'll soon get the idea.

When it comes to vegetables, fresh is always best, but tinned and frozen will work if necessary. Unless otherwise noted in a recipe, the veggies are assumed to be raw – but if you'd rather steam them, that's okay too! Chop them the way you prefer them.

As far as the dressings go, you can either make your own or use a good-quality, natural, organic shop-bought one. For added freshness, you can put the dressing in a separate little pot or keep a portable bottle of dressing to hand so you can dress the salad just before you start 'grazing'. Once you've dressed your box, remember to put the lid on and give it the 5-second tremor to mix it up.

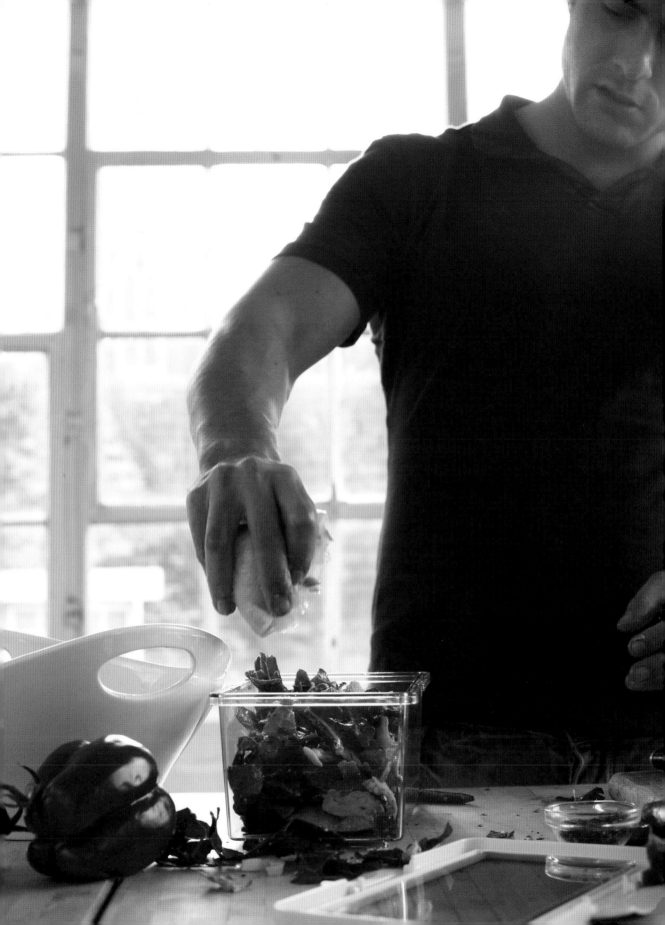

Fish
Slender Sunshine

Group A
1 beetroot
1 tomato
2 carrots
1 handful alfalfa sprouts
2 handfuls mixed dark green leaves

Group B
Cod fillet

Group C
Vinaigrette made with balsamic vinegar (see page 85)
Lemon juice to taste (probably ½ a lemon)
1tsp sunflower seeds

Active Carb option: Rye crackers

1 Cube and steam the beetroot. Chop the tomato and carrots then put all the Group A ingredients in your box.

2 Preheat your grill to moderate and grill the cod on both sides until it is slightly flaky (test it with a fork).

3 Break the cod into chunks and put it in your box, then sprinkle over the sunflower seeds, vinaigrette and squeeze the lemon juice on top.

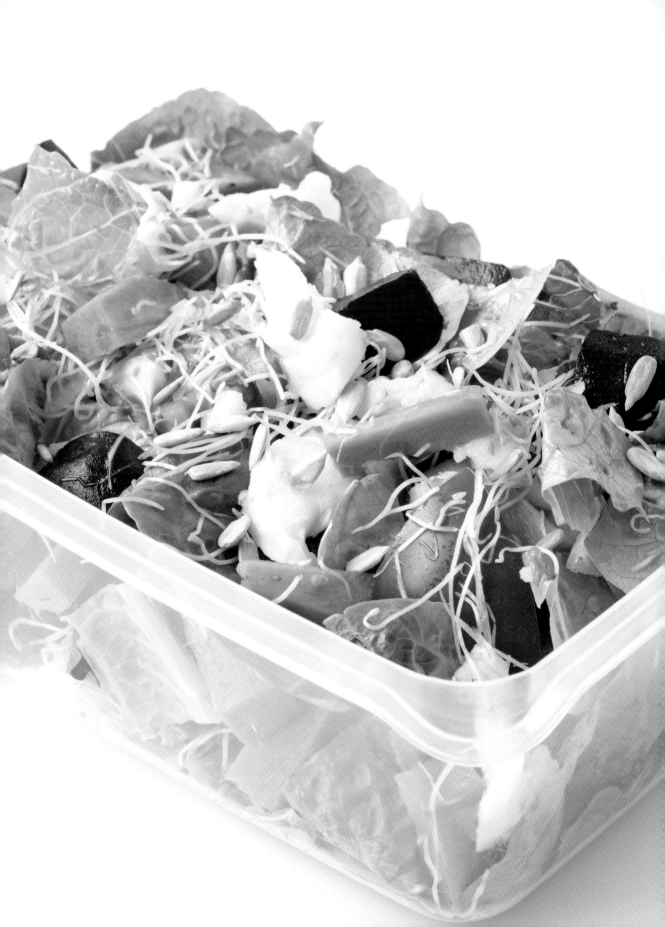

Fish
Slippery Sardine

Group A

2 handfuls lettuce

1 handful chanterelle mushrooms

12 baby carrots

12 cherry tomatoes

1 handful alfalfa sprouts

Group B

1 small tin of sardines in spring water

Group C

Raspberry vinaigrette (see page 85)

Active Carb option: Wholegrain bread

1   Toss all the veggies in the box.

2   Drain the sardines and toss them in the box.

3   Sprinkle the raspberry vinaigrette over the top.

Better Belly Bass

Group A

1 handful cauliflower

1 handful broccoli

3 stalks celery

2 carrots

2 handfuls Swiss chard

Group B

Sea bass

Group C

Home-made tzatziki (see page 214)

   or shop-bought hot pepper sauce

Fresh herbs – try dill

Active Carb option: Wholewheat pasta

1 You may steam the cauli and broccoli if you like, but raw is great too. Break them into florets, chop the celery and carrots and toss all the veggies in the box.

2 Grill the sea bass under a moderate grill, turning once, until the flesh is slightly flaky when tested with a fork. Don't overcook it – it should retain its oils. Remove the bones and flake chunks of flesh over the box.

3 Flavour with tzatziki or pepper sauce, herbs and black pepper to taste.

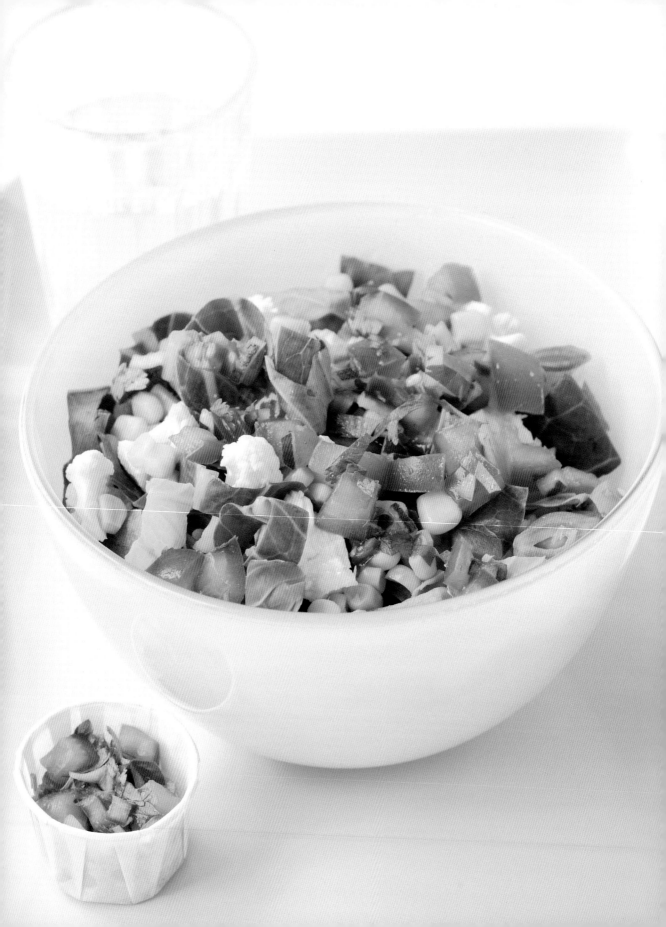

Fish
Mighty Sword

Group A
1 cup sweetcorn
1 handful cauliflower
1 handful runner beans
1 handful of dark green mixed leaves

Group B
Swordfish

Group C
2–3 tablespoons fresh salsa (see page 214)

Active Carb option: Bulgur wheat

1 Boil or microwave the sweetcorn, depending on whether you're using fresh or frozen sweetcorn. Steam the cauliflower and runner beans if you like, or leave them raw. Slice the tomato and toss all the veggies together in the box.

2 Grill the swordfish on both sides until slightly flaky but not dried out. Cut into chunks and add to the box.

3 Spoon the fresh salsa on top.

Fish

Trendy Tuna

Group A
2 leeks
½ avocado
½ red pepper
2 carrots
2 handfuls mixed spring greens

Group B
Tuna steak

Group C
Fresh lemon juice
1 tsp olive oil
Fresh parsley

Active Carb option: **Brown rice**

1 Discard the green leaves of the leeks and chop into bite-sized chunks then steam lightly. Chop the avocado, pepper and carrots and toss the veggies together in the box.

2 Grill the tuna steak lightly on both sides but leave it pink in the middle. Slice and toss in the box.

3 Whisk together the lemon juice, olive oil and shredded parsley and drizzle over the top.

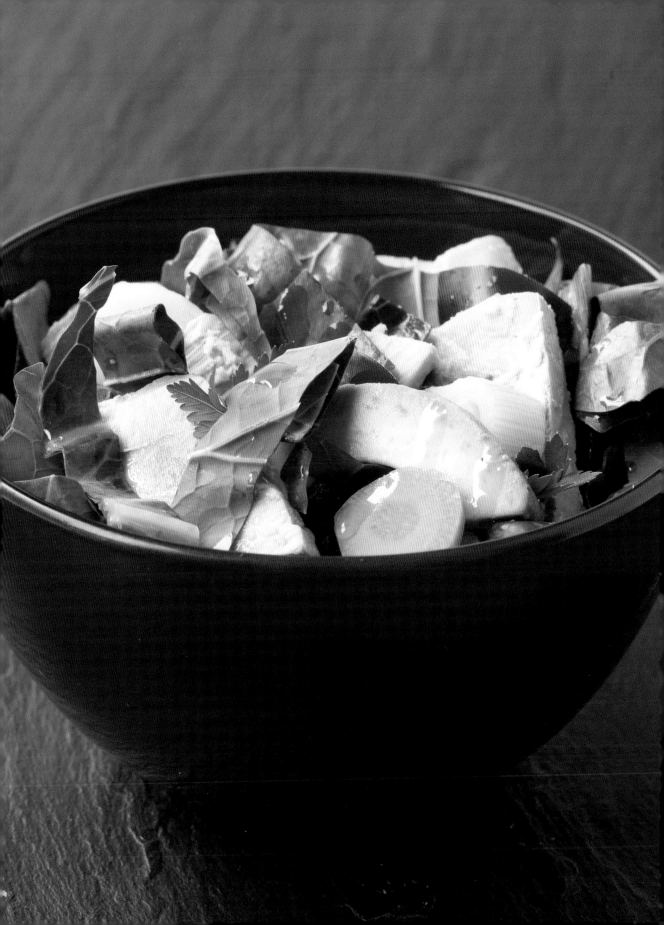

Fish
Lip-Smackin' Mack

Group A
½ avocado
1 tomato
Mixed red, green and yellow peppers (or chilli peppers)
3 or 4 spring onions
2 handfuls dark green mixed leaves

Group B
Mackerel – fillets or whole fish

Group C
Best Fish Marinade (see page 213)
Shop-bought pepper sauce, if liked

Active Carb option: **Wild rice**

1 Prepare the fish marinade and set some aside to use as dressing at the end. Using the rest, marinade the mackerel for a couple of hours before it's needed.

2 Chop the avocado and tomato and slice the peppers into strips. Trim the spring onions then toss the Group A ingredients in the box.

3 Grill the mackerel on both sides until it flakes easily. If you've used a whole fish, remove the bones. Flake the flesh into your box.

4 Sprinkle the dressing over the top and some pepper sauce to taste.

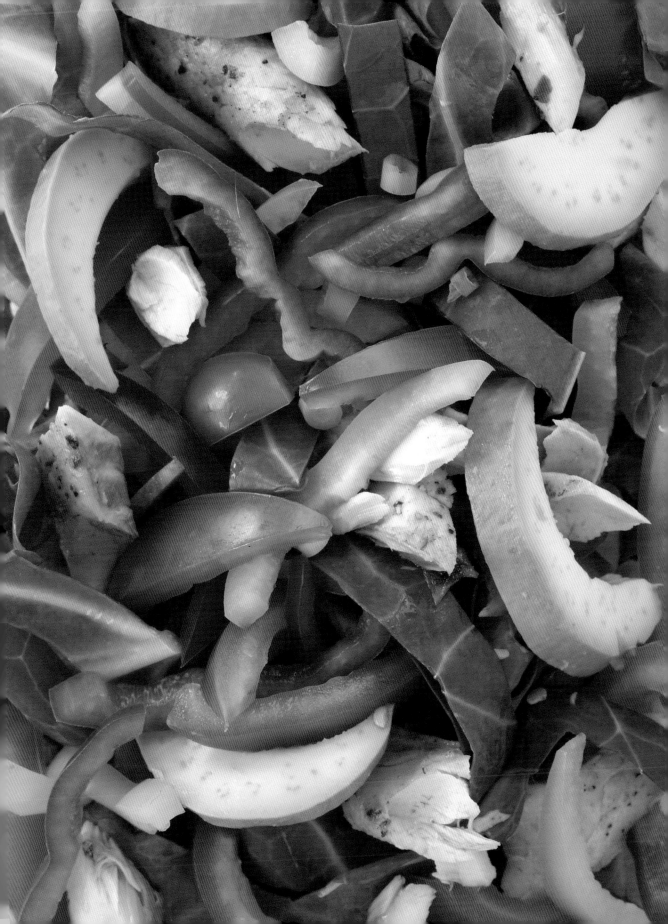

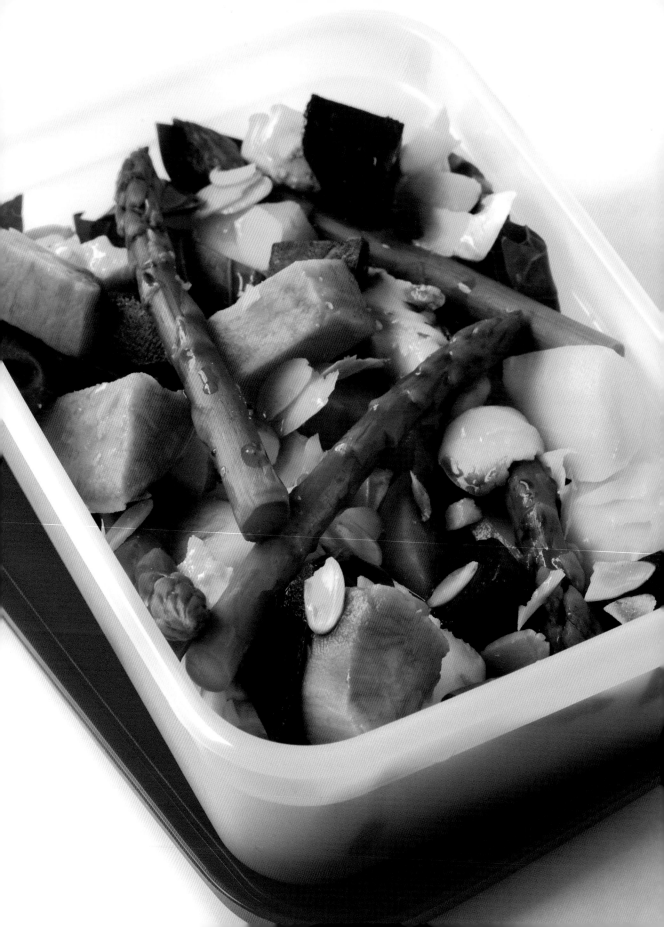

Fish
Sweet and Sour Fish

Group A
1 beetroot
1 sweet potato
1 parsnip
6 asparagus tips
2 handfuls dark green mixed leaves

Group B
Haddock fillet

Group C
Vinaigrette made with balsamic vinegar (see page 85)
1 teaspoon flaked almonds

Active Carb option: **Rye crackers**

1 Peel, cube and steam the beetroot, sweet potato and parsnip until done. Steam the asparagus slightly. Toss all the veggies in the box with the mixed leaves.

2 Grill the haddock until it flakes with a fork but is still moist. Break into chunks in the box.

3 Sprinkle balsamic vinaigrette to taste and toss the almonds on top.

Fish

Sexy Salmon

Group A

3 celery stalks
1 cucumber
1 yellow pepper
6 radishes
2 handfuls spring greens

Group B

Salmon fillets

Group C

½ cup apple chunks
1 tsp sunflower seeds
1 tsp olive oil
Juice of 1 lemon

Active Carb option: Bulgur wheat

1 Slice the celery, cucumber and pepper and put all the veggies in the box.

2 Grill the salmon fillets on both sides until the flesh flakes easily but they are definitely not dry. Cut into chunks and add to the box.

3 Sprinkle over the sunflower seeds and apple chunks and drizzle with lemon juice to taste.

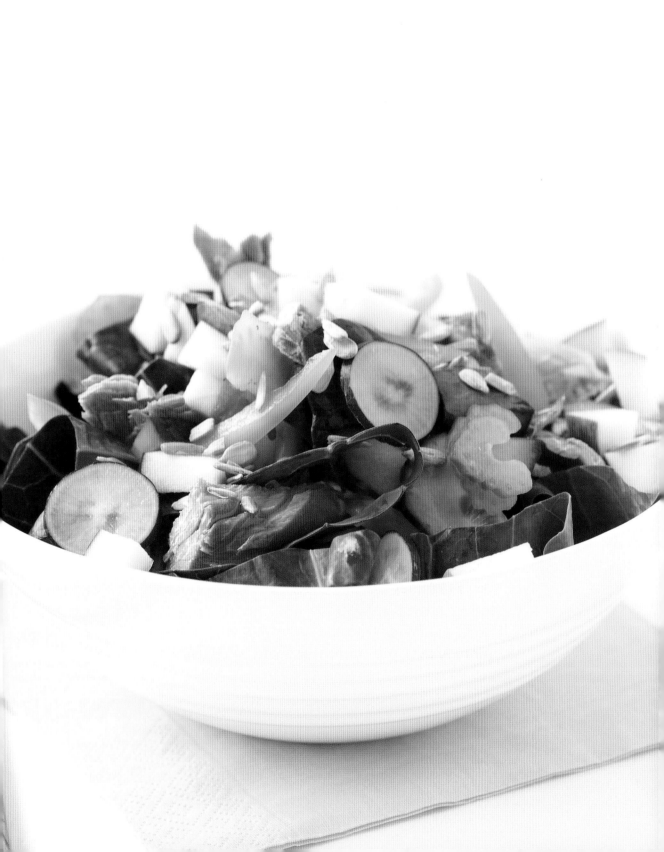

Fish
Steamy Sea

Group A
1 handful broccoli florets
1 handful sweet potato slices
1 handful brown-capped mushrooms
8 (or so) cherry tomatoes
1 handful watercress

Group B
Tuna steak

Group C
1 tsp light soy sauce
Wasabi or mustard, to taste
Grated ginger
Juice of 1 lime
1 tsp white wine vinegar

Active Carb option: Wholewheat noodles

1 Lightly steam the broccoli and sweet potatoes. Slice the mushrooms. Toss all the veggies in the box.

2 Grill the tuna steak lightly on both sides, leaving it pink in the middle. Slice and toss in the box. Alternatively, you can use a tin of tuna in spring water – drain away the water and sprinkle the tuna flakes into the box.

3 Mix the dressing ingredients together and pour over the top of your box.

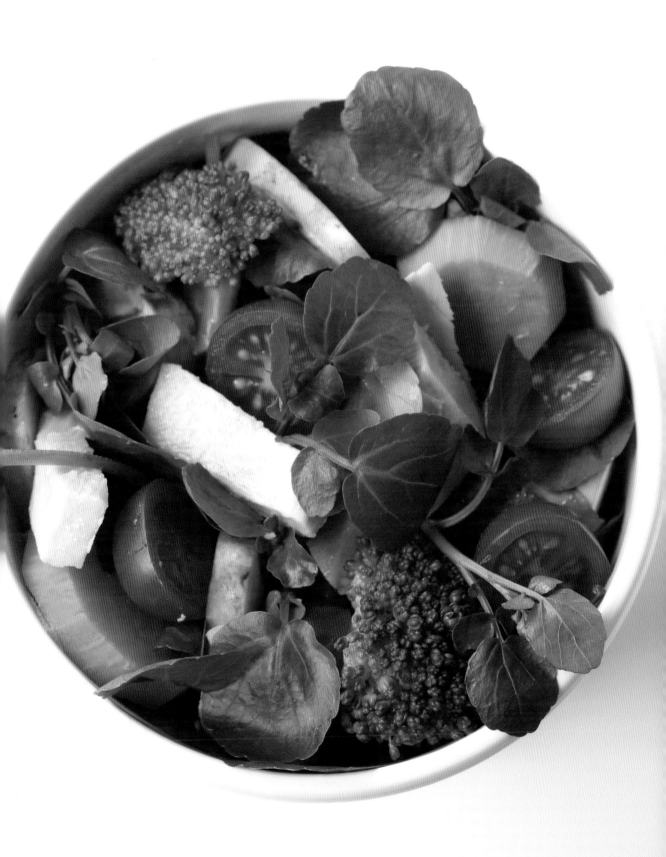

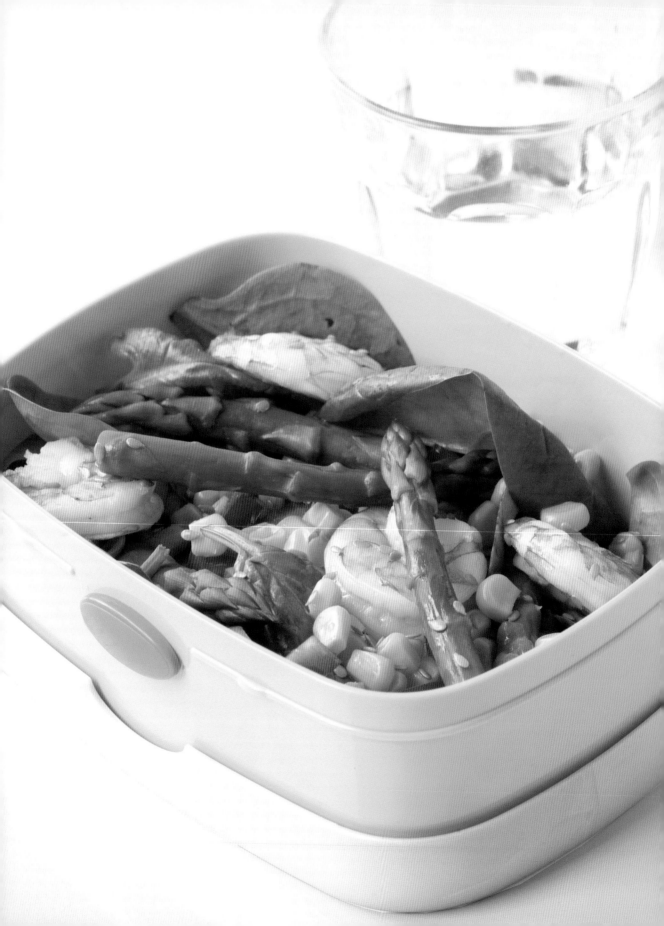

Sassy Shrimp

Group A

1 cup of sweetcorn
1 red pepper
5 asparagus tips
2 handfuls baby spinach
1 small handful mustard greens

Group B

6 king prawns

Group C

Either freshly squeezed orange juice or a shop-bought pepper sauce
1 tsp flaxseed

Active Carb option: Brown rice

1 Boil or microwave the sweetcorn, depending on whether you're using fresh or frozen sweetcorn. Dice the red pepper, lightly steam the asparagus and toss the Group A ingredients in the box.

2 Grill the prawns until they are no longer translucent and toss them in the box.

3 Sprinkle the orange juice or pepper sauce and flaxseed over the contents.

Fish
Crab Attack

Group A
1 cup sweetcorn
Small handful red onion
1 tomato
2 carrots
2 handfuls mixed dark green leaves

Group B
1 crab

Group C
Vinaigrette made with balsamic vinegar (see page 85)
or shop-bought pepper sauce

Active Carb option: **Wholegrain bread**

1 Boil or microwave the sweetcorn, depending on whether you're using fresh or frozen sweetcorn. Dice the red onion and chop the tomato and carrots then toss the veggies in the box.

2 Boil or grill the crab or buy good-quality pre-cooked crab. Shred the white and brown meat over your box. Tinned crab will work just as well.

3 Sprinkle over the vinaigrette or pepper sauce to taste.

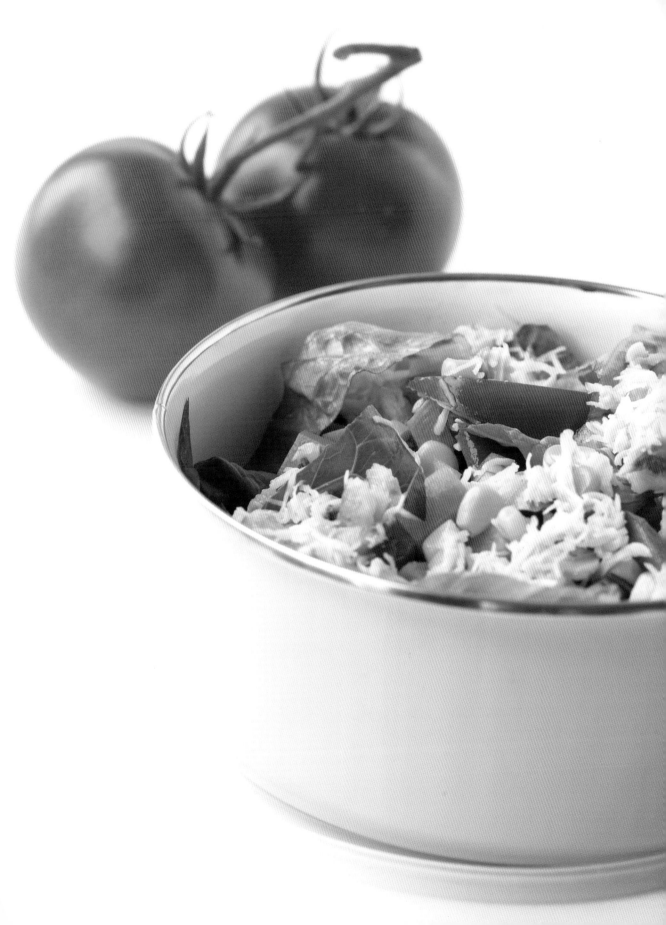

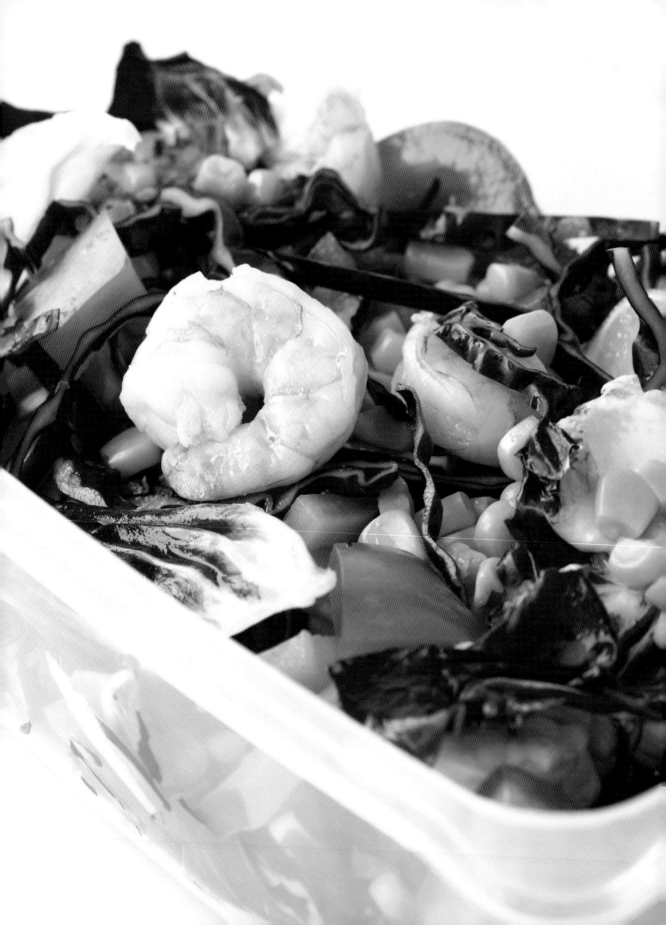

Fish
Sweet Prawn

Group A
1 cup sweetcorn
1 orange pepper
1 tomato
2 handfuls radicchio
1 handful red cabbage

Group B
6 king prawns

Group C
Lemon or lime juice
Freshly ground black pepper

Active Carb option: Wild rice

1 Boil or microwave the sweetcorn, depending on whether you're using fresh or frozen sweetcorn. Dice the pepper and tomato and shred the radicchio and cabbage, then toss all the vegetables in the box.

2 Grill the prawns until no longer translucent and place them on top of the box.

3 Sprinkle over lemon or lime juice and black pepper to taste.

Fish

Spicy Mod Cod

Group A

1 beetroot
½ courgette
2 carrots
1 handful button mushrooms
2 handfuls spring greens

Group B

Cod fillet

Group C

1 tsp Thai fish sauce
Juice of 1 lime
Shredded coriander leaves
Garlic, to taste
1 tsp flaxseed

Active Carb option: **Brown rice**

1. Cube the beetroot, slice the courgette and steam them. Chop the carrots and slice the mushrooms. Put all the veggies in the box.

2. Grill the cod until flaky but not dry, then break it into chunks in your box.

3. Mix together the Thai fish sauce, lime juice, coriander and a little crushed garlic (if using) and drizzle it over the box, followed by a sprinkling of flaxseed.

Hot Elegant Beef

Group A

12 baby carrots

6 asparagus tips

1 handful artichoke hearts

1 handful brown-capped mushrooms

1 tomato

Group B

80g lean steak

Group C

Red pepper sauce (see page 215) **or shop-bought pepper sauce**

1 tsp wholegrain mustard

Active Carb option: Wholegrain bread

1 Steam the baby carrots and asparagus tips together. Prepare the artichoke hearts by steaming and peeling the leaves of the artichokes and removing the hearts; or buy jarred artichoke hearts. Slice the mushrooms and tomato then toss all the veggies in the box.

2 Either grill the steak ahead of time or put it under the grill now for around 5 minutes on each side, depending on thickness. Cut into chunks and toss in the box.

3 Drizzle the red pepper sauce or hot pepper sauce over the top along with the mustard.

Beef
Beef Bonanza

Group A
1 handful butternut squash
5 steamed Brussels sprouts
1 handful red cabbage
1 handful portabella mushrooms
2 handfuls baby spinach

Group B
80g beef top loin

Group C
Beef Marinade (see page 212)
1 tablespoon pumpkin seeds
2 tablespoons chopped olives

Active Carb option: **Rye crackers**

1 Prepare the beef marinade and put some aside to use as dressing at the end and use the rest to marinade the beef. Cut the top loin into chunks and marinade for at least four hours.

2 Prepare the acorn squash by cubing and roasting in the oven for around 30 minutes. Steam the Brussels sprouts. Shred the red cabbage and slice the mushrooms. Warm through all the vegetables in a non-stick pan.

3 Grill the top loin chunks until cooked to your taste. Throw the vegetables then the beef into your box.

4 Sprinkle the seeds and olives on top and add the dressing that you set aside.

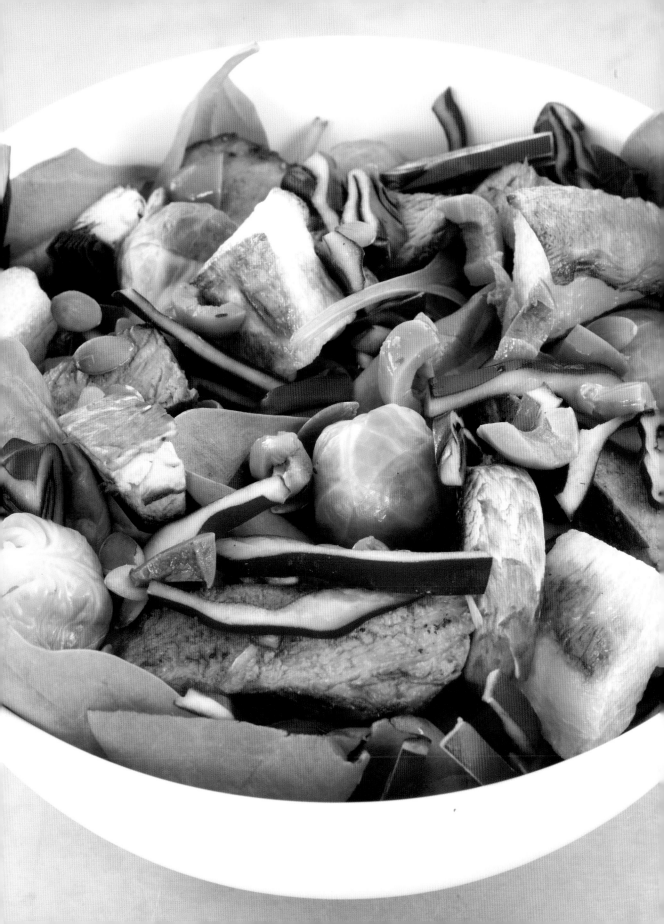

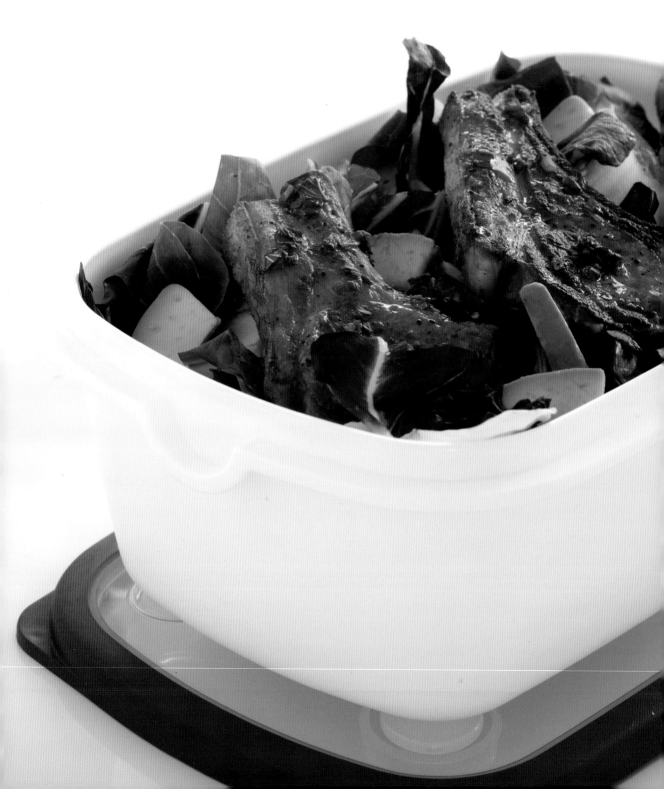

Lamb
Little Lamb

Group A

½ avocado (use the rest at supper – they don't keep long!)
½ cucumber
1 handful Swiss chard
1 handful radicchio
1 handful sugarsnap peas

Group B

2 or 3 lamb cutlets

Group C

Handful of fresh mint leaves
White wine vinegar

Active Carb option: Bulgur wheat

1 Peel and dice the avocado half. Slice the cucumber. Toss all the veggies in the box.

2 Cut off visible fat and grill the lamb cutlets. The time it takes will vary according to the thickness. Chop them into bite-sized pieces and add to the box.

3 Make a mint sauce by tearing the mint leaves and mixing them with the vinegar, then sprinkle over the top of your box.

Pork
Bashful Pork

Group A
¼ cup beetroot
1 tomato
1 handful rocket
½ dozen radishes
1 handful radicchio

Group B
80g grilled pork steaks (or leftover bits of roast pork)

Group C
Vinaigrette made with red-wine vinegar (see page 85)
1 tsp sunflower seeds

Active Carb option: **Wholewheat pasta**

1 Steam the beetroot slightly until tender and cut into chunks. Slice the tomato. Toss the veggies in the box.

2 Grill the pork steaks for about 5 minutes on each side or until they are no longer pink in the centre. Cut into chunks and toss in the box.

3 Flavour with the vinaigrette and sunflower seeds. Toss well so the dressing is evenly distributed throughout the box.

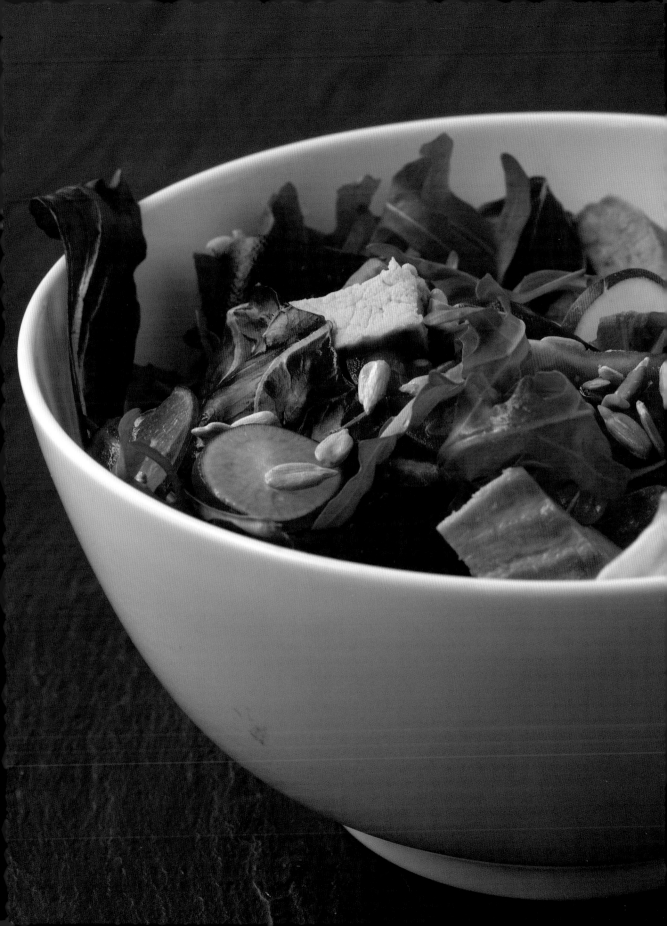

Lean Bellied Pork

Group A

1 orange pepper
1 tomato
1 cup sweetcorn
1 handful mangetout
2 handfuls spring greens

Group B

80g pork loin steaks

Group C

Peppered Pork Marinade (see page 213)
½ red onion

Active Carb option: Wholewheat noodles

1 Boil or microwave the sweetcorn, depending on whether you're using fresh or frozen sweetcorn. Slice the pepper and tomato. Mix all the veggies together in the box.

2 Prepare the Peppered Pork Marinade, setting some aside to use later as dressing. Brush the remaining marinade over the pork steaks. Grill on one side then turn over and brush on more marinade. Cook until they are no longer pink in the middle then cut them into chunks and add to the box.

3 Finely chop the red onion and sprinkle over the top. Pour over the dressing that you set aside earlier.

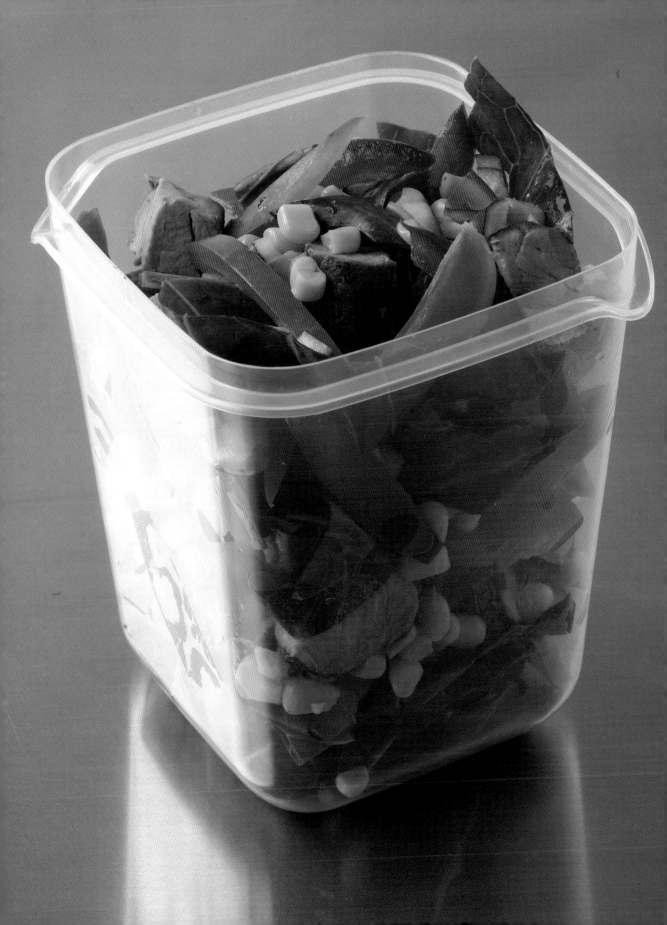

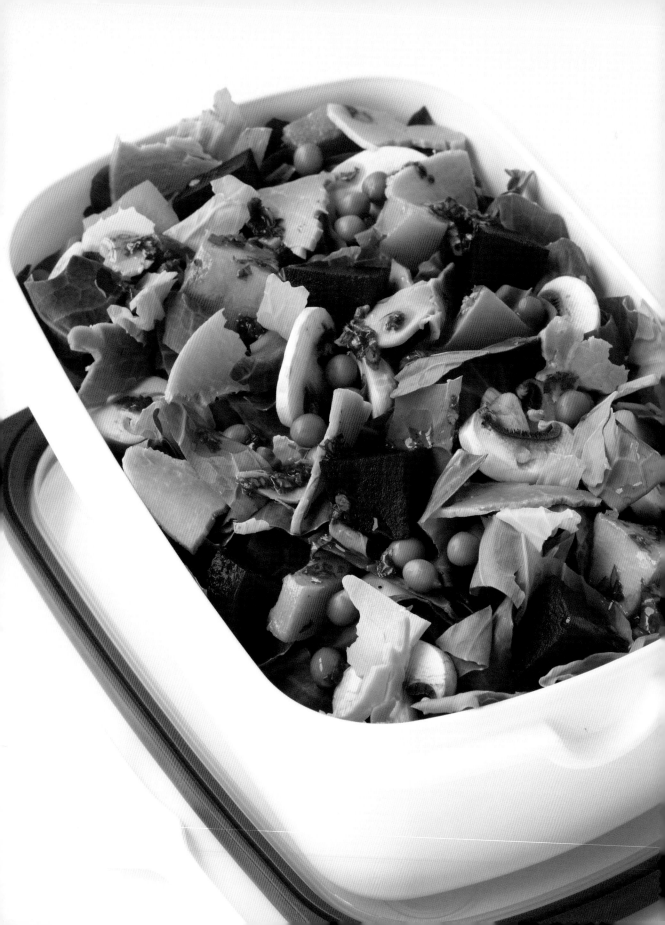

Market Ham

Group A

1 winter squash (orange)
½ beetroot
1 handful peas
1 handful button mushrooms
2 handfuls mixed spring greens

Group B

30g premium ham slices (no more – easy does it!)

Group C

Vinaigrette made with white-wine vinegar and sweet basil
(see page 85)

Active Carb option: Wholegrain bread

1   Bake the squash in the oven until soft but not mushy (about 20–30 minutes). Don't attempt to peel the hard rind from the squash until after you've cooked it. Let it cool then cube it while it's still on the rind and scrape the flesh off. Cube and bake the beetroot at the same time. Alternatively you can steam them both in a small amount of water in the microwave by cubing them and then peeling the rind after cooking. Steam the peas. Slice the mushrooms and throw the veggies in the box.

2   Cut or tear the ham into strips and add to the box.

3   Flavour the basic vinaigrette recipe with torn sweet basil leaves and drizzle over the top.

Poultry

Razzle Dazzle

Group A

5 asparagus tips
1 handful red cabbage
1 red pepper
1 tomato
2 handfuls Swiss chard

Group B

1 turkey breast or roughly 3 slices turkey from a deli

Group C

Home-made pesto sauce (see page 215)

Active Carb option: Wild rice

1   Steam the asparagus tips until slightly tender. Shred the red cabbage and dice the red pepper and tomato then toss all the veggies in the box.

2   Grill your turkey breast on both sides until it is no longer pink in the middle then cut into chunks, or buy good-quality deli meat and cut it into strips. Add them to the box.

3   Blend up all your pesto ingredients and drizzle over the top.

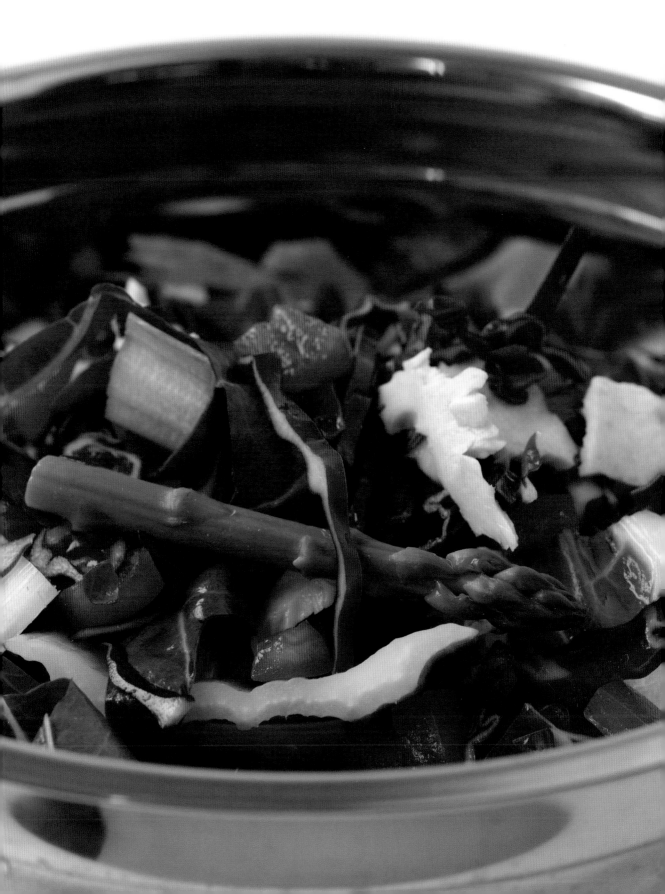

Poultry
Trim Turkey

Group A

1 cup sweetcorn
2 handfuls dark green mixed leaves
1 handful cherry tomatoes
1 cup of watermelon cubes
1 handful broccoli florets

Group B

3 slices peppered, pre-cooked turkey breast from the deli

Group C

30g feta cheese
1 teaspoon sesame seeds
Vinaigrette made with balsamic vinegar (see page 85)

Active Carb option: **Bulgur wheat**

1 If you're using fresh sweetcorn, boil a couple of cobs, let them cool slightly and shave off the kernels using a knife. Frozen organic sweetcorn is perfectly acceptable; just microwave for a minute. Throw the veggies in the box.

2 Cut the peppered turkey into strips and add it on top.

3 Crumble the feta cheese and sprinkle it on your box, along with the sesame seeds. Finish with the vinaigrette.

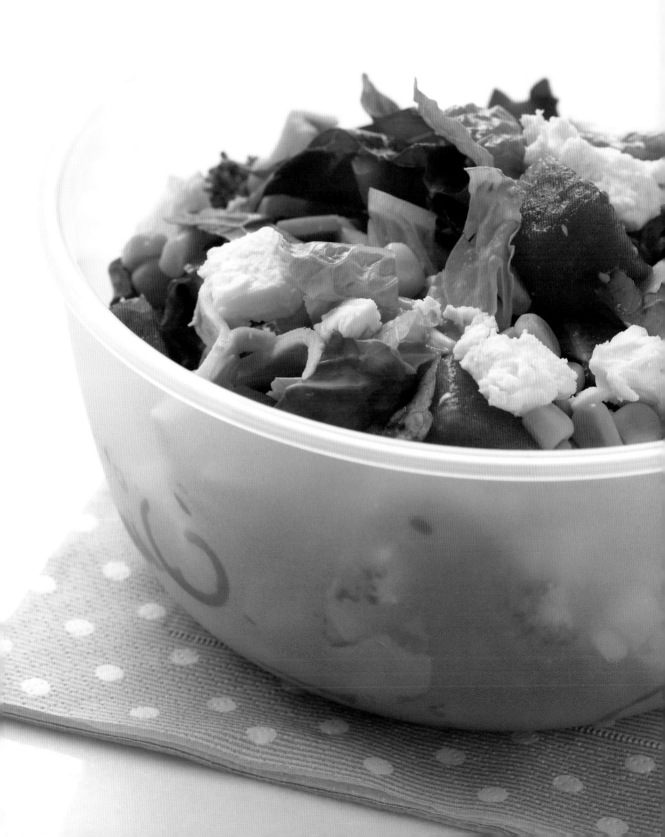

Poultry
Chicken Tango

Group A
1 handful artichoke hearts
1 small cucumber
1 handful spring greens
6 cherry tomatoes
1 handful mangetout

Group B
1 large chicken breast or roughly 3 slices pre-cooked chicken

Group C
Teriyaki Chicken Marinade (see page 213)
Mixed herbs – try chervil or tarragon
Light soy sauce

Active Carb option: **Wholewheat noodles**

1 Prepare the Teriyaki Chicken Marinade and set some aside to use as dressing. Use the rest to marinate your chicken breast overnight.

2 Prepare the artichokes by steaming them, peeling back the leaves and removing the heart. Keep the hearts and discard the rest. Alternatively, you can buy jarred artichoke hearts. Slice the cucumbers and shred the spring greens. Toss all the veggies in the box.

3 Grill your chicken breast until it is no longer pink in the middle, or use pre-cooked chicken. Slice and add to the box. Add the herbs, dressing and a sprinkle of light soy sauce.

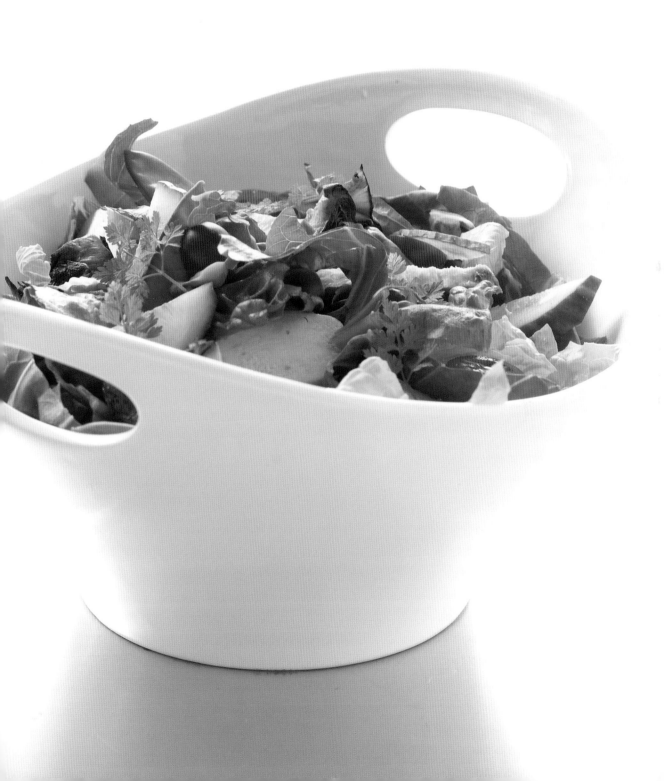

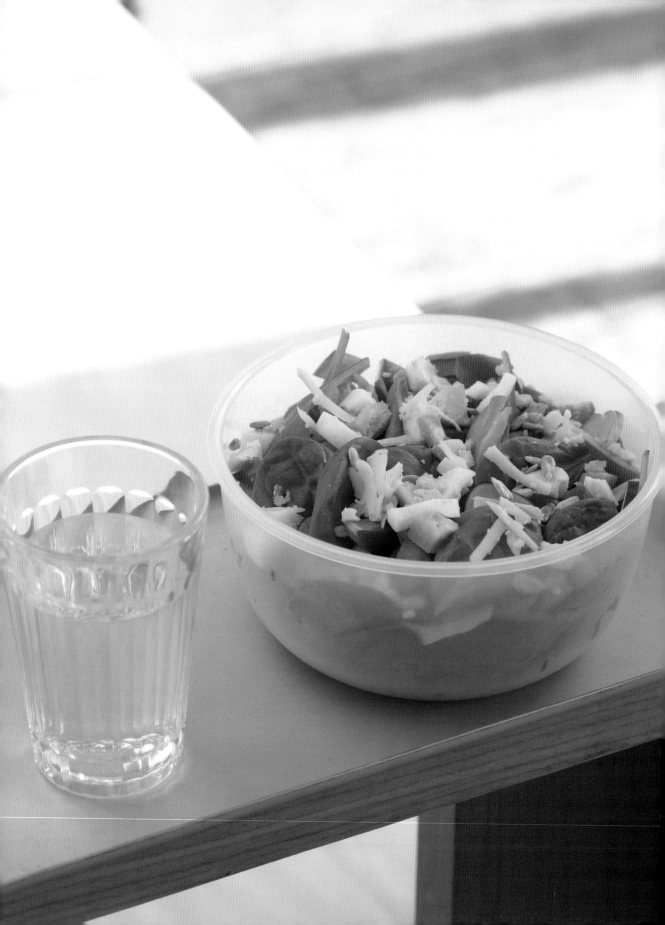

Eggs
Eggstrordinaire

Group A
1 tomato
2 carrots
2 handfuls baby spinach
1 handful oyster mushrooms
6 radishes

Group B
2 eggs

Group C
Sunflower seeds
1 tablespoon grated cheese
Vinaigrette made with balsamic vinegar (see page 85)

Active Carb option: Rye crackers

1   Dice the tomato and carrots. Toss all the veggies in the box.

2   Boil the eggs for 3 minutes and let them sit for around 20 minutes until fully cooked. Rinse them in cold water to keep the yolks nice and yellow. Peel the shells and slice the eggs.

3   Add the sunflower seeds, grated cheese and vinaigrette.

Egg
Spicy Scrambler

Group A

1 parsnip
6 asparagus tips
1 handful artichoke hearts
1 tomato
2 handfuls baby spinach

Group B

2 eggs

Group C

Shop-bought pepper sauce (green preferably)**, harissa paste or black olive tapenade.**

Active Carb option: Wholegrain bread

1 Scramble the eggs in a non-stick pan and leave to cool.

2 Cube and steam the parsnip along with the asparagus tips. Prepare the artichoke hearts by steaming and peeling the leaves of the artichokes or buy jarred artichoke hearts. Slice the tomato. Throw all the veggies together in the box.

3 Add the scrambled eggs, put the lid on and give it a shake.

4 Add the pepper sauce, harissa paste or tapenade to taste and you have a sort of breakfast scrambler in a box to munch on all day.

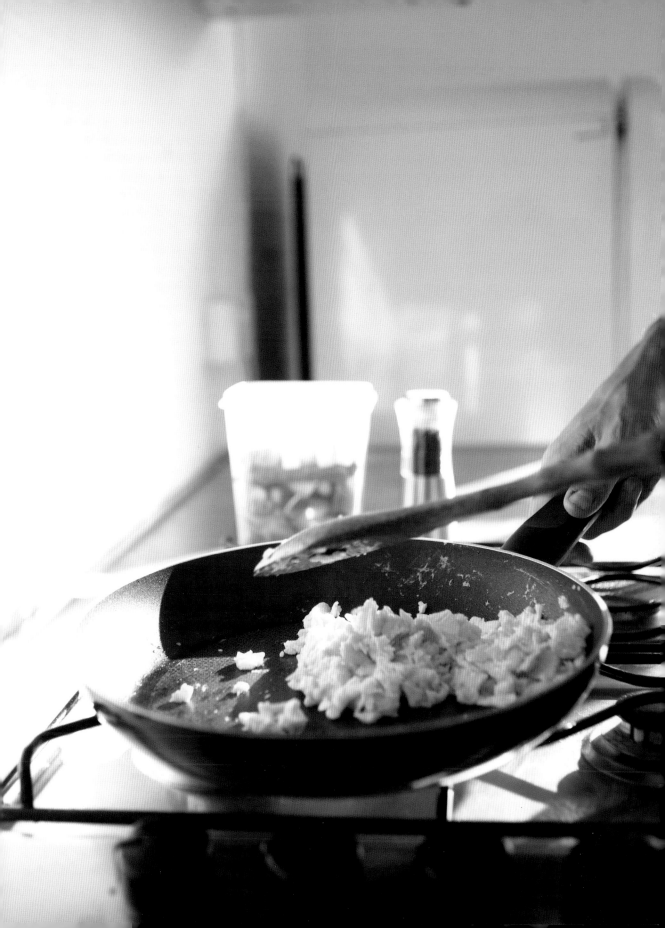

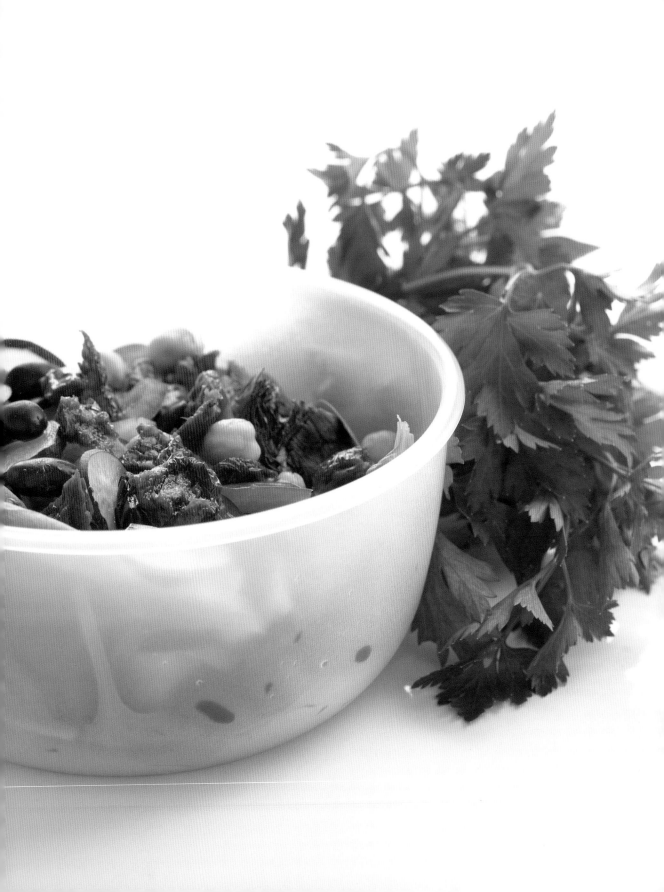

Legume I Presume?

Group A

1 handful artichoke hearts
½ green pepper
½ red onion
½ dozen radishes
2 handfuls baby spinach

Group B

½ cup kidney beans
½ cup chickpeas

Group C

Parsley
2 or 3 sundried tomatoes in olive oil
1tsp balsamic vinegar

Active Carb option: **Wild rice**

1 Steam the artichokes, peel back the leaves and remove the hearts – or to save time, buy yourself a jar of artichoke hearts. Dice the green pepper and onion. Toss all the veggies in the box.

2 Rinse the kidney beans and chickpeas and toss in the box. Flavour with a sprinkling of chopped fresh parsley, 2 or 3 sundried tomatoes cut into small pieces and a drizzle of balsamic vinegar.

Plant Proteins
Fruity Tofuti

Group A
3 slices aubergine
2 handfuls pak choi
2 carrots
1 handful baby sweetcorn
1 handful sugarsnap peas

Group B
Tofu, ready-cooked

Group C
2 tablespoons Mango Chutney (see page 214)

Active Carb option: Bulgur wheat

1 Spray the aubergine slices lightly with olive oil spray then grill them under a hot grill until tender for about 10 minutes. Steam the pak choi. Chop the carrots. Throw all the veggies in the box.

2 Cut the tofu into thin slices and add.

3 Prepare the mango chutney and dollop on top.

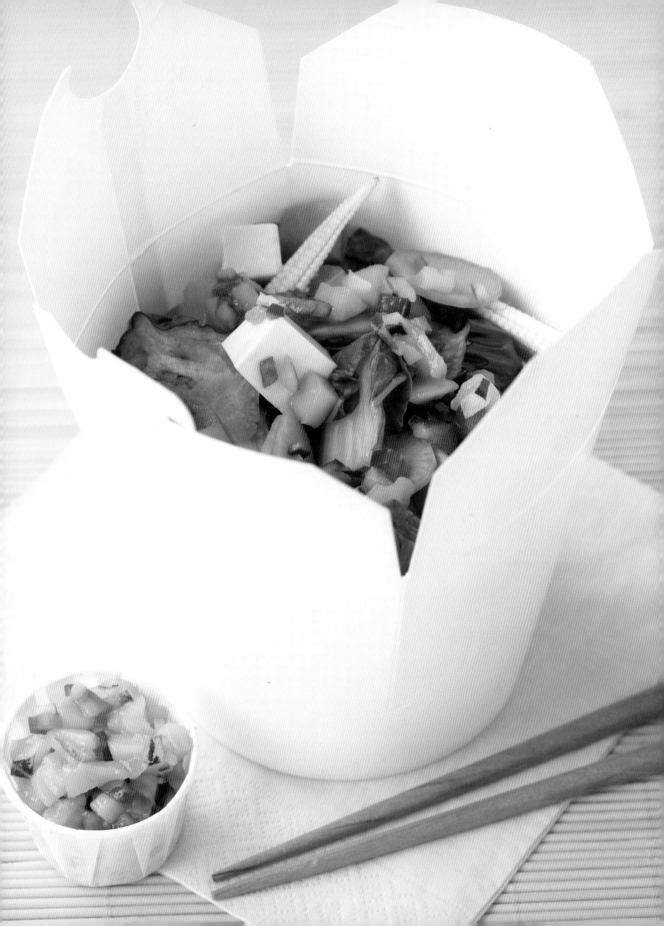

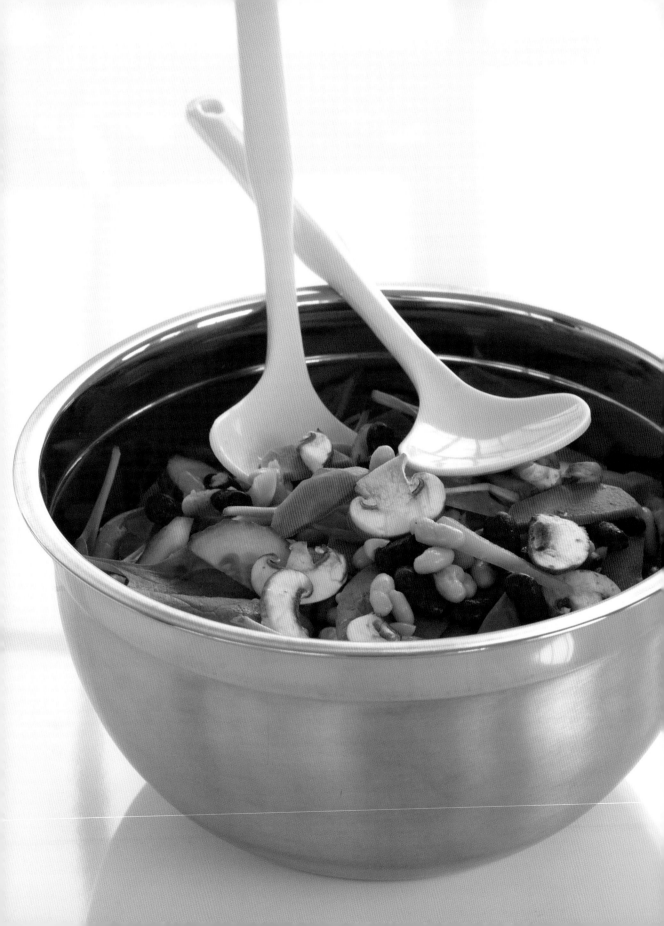

Plant Proteins

Beany Berry

Group A

1 yellow pepper
2 carrots
1 handful brown-capped mushrooms
1 small cucumber
2 handfuls baby spinach

Group B

½ tin mixed beans (kidney, flageolet, aduki
    – see what mixtures you can find)

Group C

Raspberry vinaigrette (see page 85)

Active Carb option: Wholewheat pasta

1   Chop the pepper and carrot, slice the mushrooms
    and cucumber and toss in all the veggies.

2   Rinse the beans and add them to your box.

Make a raspberry vinaigrette and pour this on at the end.

This is a super-quick box for mornings when speed is
essential.

Simon's Lunch Box Diet Marinades

These fantastic marinades can also be used as dressings. If you're making a recipe that requires the marinade, simply set some aside at the start to use later as dressing and use the rest to marinate the meat or fish.

Beef Marinade

½ **cup red wine vinegar**
1 **tsp olive oil**
1 **clove garlic, minced**
½ **red onion, finely chopped**
1 **tsp black pepper**
1 **tbsp Worcestershire sauce**

Whisk all the ingredients together.
Marinate beef for four hours.

Spicy Beef Marinade

1 **tsp olive oil**
¼ **cup soy sauce**
3 **tsp lemon juice**
1 **tsp cayenne pepper**
1 **tsp chili powder**

Whisk all the ingredients together. Marinate beef for four hours.

Peppered Pork

2 tbsp balsamic vinegar
2 tbsp soy sauce
1 tsp crushed red pepper
1 tsp chilli powder
½ tsp cayenne pepper
1 tsp black pepper

Whisk all the ingredients together. Brush over pork just before cooking.

Teriyaki Chicken Marinade

½ cup soy sauce
½ tsp honey
½ tsp grated ginger
1 tsp sesame oil
4 tbsp lemon juice
1 clove garlic, crushed
¼ red onion, chopped

Whisk all the ingredients together. Marinate chicken for two to four hours.

Best Fish Marinade

1 tsp sunflower oil
1 cup lemon juice
1 tsp black pepper
1 tsp coriander

Whisk together. Marinate fish for two hours, but be aware that it will 'cook' in this marinade.

Simon's Lunch Box Diet Dressings

Mango Chutney

1 mango, chopped
½ red onion, chopped
½ red bell pepper, chopped
1 jalapeno chilli, deseeded and chopped
Juice of 2 limes
2 tbsp wine or cider vinegar

Mix all the ingredients together and leave for a few hours to let the flavours combine before serving.

Fresh Salsa

3 vine-ripened tomatoes, chopped
1 habanero chilli pepper, deseeded and chopped
1 red onion, finely chopped
1 tbsp fresh coriander leaves
1 clove garlic, crushed
1 tsp olive oil
Juice of 2 limes

Mix together and leave for a few hours to let the flavours combine.

Tzatziki

4 tbsp natural, low-fat yoghurt
¼ cucumber, finely chopped
1 tsp lemon juice

½ clove garlic, crushed
1 tsp olive oil
1 tbsp fresh mint leaves

Mix together and store in the fridge until ready to use.

Red Pepper Sauce

1 red pepper
2 cloves garlic
1 tomato, peeled and finely chopped
1 tbsp coriander leaves
2 tsp olive oil
2 tsp lemon juice
pinch of ground cumin

Roast the pepper and garlic cloves under a hot grill until soft. Peel the peppers and chop into little pieces, and chop the garlic. Add the other ingredients and mix well (or blitz in a blender for a smoother sauce). Leave for a few hours to let the flavours combine.

Fresh Pesto

1 handful fresh basil leaves
2 tsp freshly grated Parmesan
2 tsp olive oil
2 tbsp pine nuts
1 clove garlic, crushed

The old-fashioned way is to grind all the ingredients together with a mortar and pestle – but it's much easier to use a mixer! Whizz it all up and serve.

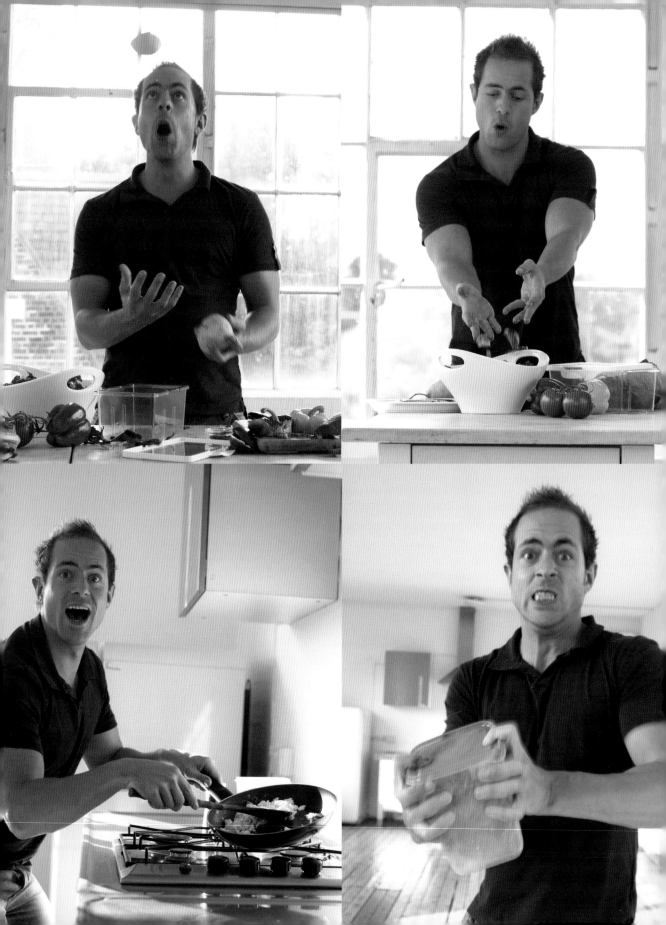

Signing off

In closing, I want to wish you all the best and thank you for buying this book. Let me know what you think of it via my website and don't forget to join the Lunch Box Diet community for continuous motivational advice! Write in and let me know about your own lunch box recipes and how things are working for you at support@lunchboxdiet.co.uk.

I hope you all lose the weight you want to and arrive at a healthier new you. I started designing this diet with weight loss for my clients in mind, hence the name the Lunch Box Diet, but as you'll soon realise it's much more than a diet. It's a revolutionary new way to eat that is effective for weight loss and creating overall good health. It fits the needs of just about anyone, no matter what their lifestyle. Pass it along to friends and family.

For now, leave me with a smile!

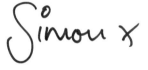

Vitamins

Vitamin A (retinol)

Function: strong bones, healthy skin, good eyesight, healing and resistance to infection

Found in: eggs, butter, fish oils, liver and as beta-carotene in dark green and yellow/orange fruits and vegetables

Vitamin B1 (thiamin)

Function: growth, nerve function, conversion of blood sugar into energy

Found in: wholegrain products, brown rice, seafood, beans, sunflower seeds, Brazil nuts, yeast extract

Vitamin B2 (riboflavin)

Function: cell growth and reproduction, energy production, healthy skin

Found in: milk and dairy products, green leafy vegetables, liver, kidneys, yeast, almonds, mushrooms, avocados

Vitamin B3 (niacin)

Function: digestion, energy production, the nervous system

Found in: meat, fish and poultry, wholegrains, peanuts, mushrooms, yeast extract, sesame seeds

Vitamin B5 (pantothenic acid)

Function: many roles including cell metabolism and synthesis of molecules

Found in: organ meats, fish, eggs, chicken, nuts and wholegrain cereals

Vitamin B6 (pyridoxine)

Function: production of antibodies and white blood cells, a healthy immune system

Found in: eggs, wholegrain products, yeast, cabbage, melon, molasses, bananas, hazelnuts

Vitamin B12 (cyanocobalamin)

Function: energy production and concentration, production of red blood cells, healthy nervous system, growth in children

Found in: fish, dairy produce, beef, pork, lamb, organ meats, eggs and milk, fortified soya milk, yeast extract

Folic acid (folate)

Function: production of new cells (working with vitamin B12), important during pregnancy to help prevent birth defects

Found in: fruit, green leafy vegetables, nuts, pulses, yeast extract

Biotin (Vitamin B7)

Function: energy production and healthy skin, hair and nails

Found in: milk, liver, egg yolk, yeast extract, pulses, nuts, most vegetables

Vitamin C (ascorbic acid)

Function: healing, protection from viruses, healthy skin, bones, muscles, teeth and eyesight

Found in: fresh fruit and vegetables, leafy herbs and berries

Vitamin D

Function: healthy teeth and bones, vital for growth

Found in: milk and dairy products, eggs, oily fish; also produced by the action of sunlight on skin

Vitamin E

Function: absorption of iron and essential fatty acids, slowing the ageing process, increasing fertility

Found in: nuts, seeds, eggs, milk, wholegrains, leafy green vegetables, avocados, soya, vegetable oils

Vitamin K

Function: for effective blood clotting

Found in: green vegetables, milk products, apricots, wholegrains, cod liver oil

Minerals

Calcium
Function: strong bones and teeth, muscle contraction, blood clotting, regulation of blood pressure, hormone regulation
Found in: dairy produce, leafy green vegetables, salmon, nuts, root vegetables, tofu, fortified soya milk

Iron
Function: supply of oxygen to the cells, healthy immune system
Found in: red meat, liver, kidney, dark chocolate, shellfish, pulses, dark green vegetables, egg yolks, molasses, pumpkin seeds and dried fruit

Magnesium
Function: transmission of nerve impulses, development of bones, growth and repair of cells
Found in: green leafy vegetables, brown rice, soya beans, nuts, wholegrains, bitter chocolate, legumes

Potassium
Function: maintaining water balance, nerve and muscle function
Found in: avocados, leafy green vegetables, bananas, fruit and vegetable juices, potatoes, wholegrain cereals and nuts

Chromium
Function: stimulating insulin to maintain blood sugar levels
Found in: liver, wholegrains, meat and cheese, mushrooms, egg yolk, black pepper

Iodine
Function: keeping hair, skin, nails and teeth healthy, production of thyroid hormones which are important for metabolism
Found in: fish and seafood, seaweed, dairy produce

Phosphorus
Function: along with calcium, it helps to keep bones and teeth strong, aids muscles function
Found in: dairy products, meat, fish, wholegrains, lentils, nuts

Sodium
Function: maintains water balance, controlling the composition of body fluids like blood
Found in: processed foods, small amounts in vegetables, fruits and grains; most people consume too much in the form of sodium chloride (salt)

Zinc
Function: involved in enzyme regulation, essential for growth and reproduction
Found in: shellfish, red meat, poultry, beans, nuts, sesame and pumpkin seeds

Copper
Function: formation of red blood cells, enzyme regulation
Found in: green vegetables, yeast, nuts, wheatgerm, offal

Selenium
Function: effective functioning of red blood cells, and has anti-ageing properties
Found in: Brazil nuts, red meat, fish, eggs, wholegrain bread, seafood, kidney

Fluorine
Function: strong bones and teeth
Found in: fluoridated water, tea, fish

Manganese
Function: aids many enzymes and helps muscle function
Found in: tea, green vegetables, wholegrain cereals, nuts, spices

Molybdenum
Function: helps certain enzymes to function
Found in: peas, leafy vegetables, cauliflower, nuts, oats

Index

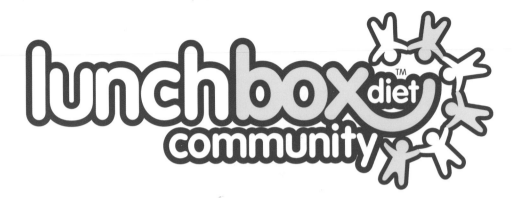

Now you've learned how the Lunch Box Diet can literally change your life, it's time to get connected to the Lunch Box Diet community – your place to share, experience, learn and make new friends on the way!

Sign up today and you can:

- Create your own profile
- View videos and listen to Simon's audio seminars
- Upload pictures, video and audio
- Start your own weight-loss blog
- Chat live with other dieters
- Get even more Lunch Box Diet combinations
- Make new friends and motivate each other

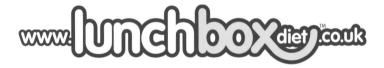

I'll see you in there!

Simon x